DISCARDED

D1445198

The Doctor of Nursing Practice and Clinical Nurse Leader

Joyce J. Fitzpatrick, PhD, MBA, RN, FAAN, is the Elizabeth Brooks Ford Professor of Nursing, Frances Payne Bolton School of Nursing, Case Western Reserve University, in Cleveland, Ohio, where she was dean from 1982 through 1997. She has received numerous honors and awards, including the *American Journal of Nursing* Book of the Year Award 18 times. Dr. Fitzpatrick is widely published in nursing and health care literature. From 1993 to 2008, she was senior editor of the *Annual Review of Nursing Research,* now in its 26th volume. In 1998, Dr. Fitzpatrick was senior editor of the first volume of the classic *Encyclopedia of Nursing Research* as well as a series of Research Digests, including *Nursing Research Digest, Maternal Child Health Nursing Research Digest, Geriatric Nursing Research Digest,* and *Psychiatric Mental Health Nursing Research Digest.* She has coedited four books focused on nurses and the Internet: *Nurses Guide to Consumer Health Web Sites* (2001), *Essentials of Internet Use in Nursing* (2002), *Internet Resources for Nurses, 2nd edition* (2003), and *Internet for Nursing Research* (2004). Dr. Fitzpatrick has provided consultation on nursing education and research throughout the world, including universities and health ministries in Africa, Asia, Australia, Europe, Latin America, and the Middle East.

Meredith Wallace, PhD, APRN-BC, completed her BSN degree Magna Cum Laude at Boston University. Following this, she earned an MSN in medical-surgical nursing with a specialty in geriatrics from Yale University, and a PhD in nursing research and theory development at New York University. During her time at NYU she was awarded a predoctoral fellowship at the Hartford Institute for Geriatric Nursing. In this capacity, she became the original author and editor of *Try This: Best Practices in Geriatric Nursing* series. In 2001, she won the Springer Publishing Company Award for Applied Nursing Research. She was the Managing Editor of the journal of *Applied Nursing Research* and is currently on the editorial board for the journal.

As noted author, educator, and researcher, her most recent books include, *Essentials of Gerontological Nursing* and *Gerontological Nurse Certification Review,* the latter with Shelia Grossman, published in 2008. Dr. Wallace is the recipient of two American Journal of Nursing Book of the Year Awards, most recently in 2007 for her work, as associate editor, on the *Encyclopedia of Nursing Research, 2nd Edition,* with Joyce Fitzpatrick, and in 2003 for *Prostate Cancer: Nursing Assessment, Management & Care,* with Lorrie Powel. Dr. Wallace is a 2007 recipient of the American Cancer Society Travel Scholarship and a 2003 recipient of the Eastern Nursing Research Society/John A. Hartford Foundation junior investigator award. She is an adult nurse practitioner and currently maintains a practice in primary care with a focus on chronic illness in the elderly along with her appointment as Associate Professor, Yale School of Nursing, New Haven, CT. Her research interests focus on the psychosocial needs of men with prostate cancer, especially those undergoing active surveillance.

The Doctor of Nursing Practice and Clinical Nurse Leader

Essentials of Program Development and Implementation for Clinical Practice

JOYCE J. FITZPATRICK, PhD, MBA, RN, FAAN
MEREDITH WALLACE, PhD, APRN-BC

Editors

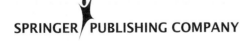

SPRINGER PUBLISHING COMPANY

New York

Springer Publishing Company, LLC
11 West 42nd Street
New York, NY 10036
www.springerpub.com

Acquisitions Editor: Allan Graubard
Production Editor: Julia Rosen
Cover design: Mimi Flow
Composition: Apex CoVantage

08 09 10 11 12/ 5 4 3 2 1

Library of Congress Cataloging-in-Publication Data

The doctor of nursing practice and clinical nurse leader : essentials of program development and implementation for clinical practice / [edited by] Joyce J. Fitzpatrick, Meredith Wallace.
      p. ; cm.
   Includes bibliographical references and index.
   ISBN 978-0-8261-3828-6 (alk. paper)
   1. Nursing—Study and teaching (Graduate)—United States.   2. Doctor of philosophy degree—United States.   3. Nurse practitioners—Education—United States.   I. Fitzpatrick, Joyce J., 1944–   II. Wallace, Meredith.
   [DNLM: 1. Education, Nursing, Graduate—United States.   2. Clinical Medicine—education—United States.   3. Nurse Clinicians—education—United States.   4. Program Development—methods—United States.   WY 18.5 D6365 2008]

   RT75.D55   2008
   610.73071'173—dc22   2008024567

Printed in the United States of America by Bang Printing.

Contents

Contributors

Linda Thompson Adams, DrPH, RN, FAAN
Dean and Professor
Oakland University
School of Nursing
Rochester, Michigan

Marianne Baernholdt, PhD, MPH, RN
Assistant Professor
University of Virginia
School of Nursing
Charlottesville, Virginia

Jean Demartinis, PhD, ARNP, FNP, PC
Associate Professor
Director, Doctor of Nursing
Practice, Clinical Nurse
Leader (CNL) Programs
University of Massachusetts
School of Nursing
Amherst, Massachusetts

Pamela D. Dennison, MSN, RN, ACNS-BC, CNL
Advanced Practice Nurse
Clinician Educator
University of Virginia Health System
Charlottesville, VA

Moreen Donahue, DNP, RN, CNA-BC
Chief Nurse Executive
Senior Vice President
Patient Care Services
Danbury Hospital
Danbury, Connecticut

Sandra E. Fox, MSN, CNL
Clinical Nurse Leader
Veteran's Administration
Tennessee Valley Healthcare
System
Nashville, Tennessee

Helen A. Gordon, MS, RN, CNM
Associate Clinical Professor
Duke University
School of Nursing
Durham, North Carolina

Sheila Grossman, PhD, FNP, APRN, BC
Professor
Fairfield University
School of Nursing
Fairfield, Connecticut

James L. Harris, DSN, APRN-BC, MBA, CNL
Program Director, Leadership
Development
Veteran's Administration
Office of Nursing Services
Washington, District of Columbia

Elizabeth A. Henneman, PhD, RN, CCNS
Associate Professor
University of Massachusetts
School of Nursing
Amherst, Massachusetts

Frances Jackson, PhD, RN
Director, Doctor of Nursing
  Practice Degree Program
Oakland University
School of Nursing
Rochester, Michigan

Jean Lange, PhD, RN, CNL
Associate Professor
Fairfield University
School of Nursing
Fairfield, Connecticut

Colleen A. Maykut, MN, RN
Doctor of Nursing Practice (c)
Faculty
Grant MacEwan College
School of Nursing
Edmonton, Alberta, Canada

Paula Miller, MSN, CNL
Clinical Nurse Leader
Veteran's Administration
Tennessee Valley Healthcare System
Nashville, Tennessee

**Ann L. O'Sullivan, PhD,
FAAN, CRNP**
Professor of Primary Care
  Nursing—Clinician Educator
University of Pennsylvania
School of Nursing
Philadelphia, Pennsylvania

Mary T. Quinn Griffin, PhD, RN
Assistant Professor
Case Western Reserve University
School of Nursing
Cleveland, Ohio

**Kathryn Reid, PhD, RN,
CCRN, C-FNP**
Assistant Professor
Director, Clinical Nurse Leader
  (CNL) Program
University of Virginia
School of Nursing
Charlottesville, Virginia

Joan Roche, PhD, RN, GCNS-BC
Clinical Assistant Professor,
  Director, Clinical Nurse Leader
  (CNL) Program
University of Massachusetts
School of Nursing
Amherst, Massachusetts

Kerri Schuiling, PhD, RN, CNM
Associate Dean for Nursing
  Education
Northern Michigan University
School of Nursing
Marquette, Michigan

**Cheryl Stegbauer, PhD,
FNP, APRN-BC**
Professor and Associate Dean for
  Academic Programs
College of Nursing
University of Tennessee Health
  Science Center
Memphis, Tennessee

June A. Treston, MSN, CRNP, RN
Associate Program Director,
Family Health Nurse
  Practitioner Program
University of Pennsylvania
School of Nursing
Philadelphia, Pennsylvania

Victoria A. Weill, MSN, CRNP
Associate Program Director
Primary Care-Pediatric Nurse
  Practitioner Program
University of Pennsylvania
School of Nursing
Philadelphia, Pennsylvania

Foreword

For almost a decade, the American Association of Colleges of Nursing (AACN) has led a series of strategic discussions and policy formulations related to the dramatically evolving nature of the health care environment and the unique contributions that nursing makes. This national dialogue has included a wide array of stakeholders from education—both nursing and higher education at large—and practice arenas. Representatives of other health professions have also contributed to this conversation.

Out of these important discussions have come two very significant and groundbreaking innovations for nursing, which this book describes: the development of the Clinical Nurse Leader (CNL®) role and the recommendation that education for advanced nursing practice should occur through professional doctoral programs that award the Doctor of Nursing Practice (DNP).

The movement toward these two innovations was framed by an understanding that health care has become increasingly complex, and that despite the sophistication of the interventions used to assure a healthy population, multiple errors and inequalities in care delivery persist. Moreover, the rapid aging of the U.S. population, the growth in diversity among patients, and the enhanced application of technology both for patient care and information management have created a need for an increasingly competent nursing professional.

The need for the CNL emerged from the work of nurse executives to apply positive deviance theory and design a new nursing role that would focus on the clinical microsystem, evidence-based practice, the outcomes of care, and how the interprofessional health care team can collaborate to unify fragmented care. These nurse executives urged AACN to lead in the development of a new model of education to create a highly competent generalist clinician with the ability to address all these issues. The work of two AACN task forces—the Task Force on Education and Regulation for Professional Nursing Practice I and II—responded to this call with the recommendation that AACN support the creation of master's degree-educated advanced generalist nurses who would fill the CNL role.

To support this evolution in professional nursing, AACN sought teams of education and practice partners who would lead in this national experiment. The overwhelming response in which more than 100 academic nursing programs and almost 200 clinical partners joined AACN to implement this innovation provides evidence that the role is filling a much needed void in the health care system. The continued expansion and support for this work in multiple arenas including the largest nursing system in the US, the Department of Veteran's Affairs, gives further evidence that the CNL is needed to fulfill the professional mandate to provide high quality and safe patient care.

The movement to the DNP is focused on the education for advanced nursing practice, including nurse specialists engaged in providing a full array of health care services. The approval of the AACN position statement on the DNP by institutional members in 2004 was the culmination of similar work in which stakeholders from practice, education, other health professions, and policy makers at large discussed and framed the challenges facing nurses functioning at the highest possible level. The challenges being faced by entry level and advanced generalist nursing clinicians are also part of the framework of advanced nursing practice. Further, the educational programs that prepared advanced nursing clinicians had for some time been reformulating curriculum to address the growing need for expanded knowledge and competencies for specialized practice.

The Task Force on the Practice Doctorate in Nursing reviewed the shifting nature of advanced nursing education curricula and noted that these programs carried credit loads that exceeded the norm for master's degree in other professional fields. Further, both clinicians and employers identified the need for these advanced nursing professionals to have exposure to other content that was not traditionally included in the master's level programs such as aggregate data management, translational science, analysis of costs and outcomes of care, identification of evidence gaps, and formulations of system level interventions and monitoring. Coincident with the work of the AACN task force, the National Academy of Science released a report on the future research workforce for all health professions and recommended that nursing develop two distinct pathways to the terminal degree, thus allowing nursing professionals to make decisions about whether to pursue a research-focused or practice-focused degree.

Similar to the very positive response to the CNL, AACN has witnessed a dramatic and rapid uptake of the recommendations in the DNP position statement with new programs emerging monthly. The target recommendation to transition to the DNP from the master's degree for the education of advanced specialized nursing clinicians by 2015 is widely accepted, and work continues in many communities including accreditation, certification, and regulation.

AACN is committed to supporting innovation in nursing education and practice to assure that our nation is served by expert clinicians delivering high quality and safe professional nursing care. We look forward to continued expansion of these two innovations and trust that AACN will continue to lead in these efforts.

C. Fay Raines, PhD, RN
Geraldine "Polly" Bednash, PhD, RN, FAAN

—Dr. Fay Raines, President (2008-2010)
American Association of Colleges of Nursing

Dr. Geraldine Bednash, Executive Director
American Association of Colleges of Nursing

Preface

This book is a direct result of the editors' firm commitment to advanced education for nurses in clinical practice. Throughout my career in nursing education I have supported the professional doctorate. In 1990 with faculty colleagues I implemented the first post-master's clinical doctoral program at Case Western Reserve University (Case). We were anxious to lead the revolution for nursing education and demonstrate the excellence of our students and graduates. Since that time, and even preceding the Case program implementation, there have been scholarly deliberations at educational conferences and debates in the literature regarding the best approach for nursing education, particularly for those nurses functioning at the highest levels of clinical practice.

When the American Association of Colleges of Nursing (AACN) launched its planning effort for the professional doctorate we at Case were ecstatic, as we considered this a "tipping point" for the movement toward advanced education for nurses in clinical practice. The strength of the Doctor of Nursing Practice (DNP) movement as we know it today is evidence that the nursing education and professional practice communities were ready for the change. Within a short period of time after the introduction of the DNP, AACN also launched the Clinical Nurse Leader (CNL) program initiative.

In this book, my coeditor, Meredith Wallace, and I have profiled these historical changes in nursing education. We have selected contributors who have been involved in the DNP and CNL movements from several perspectives, from architects of the programs to those who are students in selected programs. This book is intended as an introduction to the two programs, prepared as a marker of a point in time, when there have been proposed program designs. Yet, we know that the evolution will continue and that the development of DNP and CNL program objectives, curricula, and expected outcomes are not static.

One of the most important contributions of this book is charting the development of doctoral education in nursing, from its earliest roots at

Teachers College, Columbia University, to the current DNP programs development at several top universities. Chapters 1 through 3 set the foundation for consideration of the current status of DNP programs. Chapters 4 and 5 identify important issues for future DNP program development, including the impact on the clinical environment for the student and the graduate.

Chapters 6 through 9 include particular attention to the historical development of the CNL programs. Authors delineate the core program requirements and the expectations of students and graduates in the clinical and academic arenas. Particularly important is the discussion of the transition of current master's-level nursing education programs to the CNL program.

There are several other components of this book that are important contributions to the state of the art of nursing education regarding the DNP and CNL. The critical issues of credentialing, certification, and licensure of graduates are addressed in Chapter 10. Chapters 11 and 12 include "voices from the field" of current DNP and CNL students. These voices add a dimension that could not be garnered from the program designers or faculty and thus present a different perspective.

We are particularly indebted to AACN for granting permission for the inclusion of several documents related to the DNP and CNL programs. These inclusions again will serve to mark a "point in time" and will assist those who are in the process of program design to obtain all of the relevant materials in one place.

We are hopeful regarding future developments for graduate education in nursing, particularly for the preparation of nurse clinicians at the same level as colleagues in other health disciplines. It is extremely satisfying to witness the unfolding of a professional dream, that of doctoral education for advanced clinical practice in nursing. It also is most rewarding to share information about the dream unfolding in this book. We, the editors and chapter authors, know that this work will stir continued discussion and debate.

Joyce J. Fitzpatrick, PhD, MBA, RN, FAAN
Editor

History of Graduate Nursing Education

JOYCE J. FITZPATRICK

Nursing education at all levels has had a multifaceted history, and so it is with graduate education, at both the master's and doctoral levels. Whereas in many disciplines and professions there are straightforward paths to both academic degrees and professional credentialing, in nursing, both historically and currently, there exist a myriad of educational options. The diversity of entry and exit points in nursing education is confusing to the public and often also difficult for those in other health professions to understand. The focus of this book is on two new educational pathways in nursing, the Doctor of Nursing Practice (DNP) and the Clinical Nurse Leader (CNL®). Yet, it is important to frame this presentation within the context of both the broader educational issues in nursing and the societal context.

BASIC EDUCATION FOR NURSING

There are four paths for entering nursing and four for exiting nursing education at the prelicensure level. Students can enter associate degree (AD) programs (offered primarily through community colleges), diploma programs (offered through hospital schools of nursing), baccalaureate programs (offered through colleges and universities) and graduate-level entry programs (offered through colleges and universities, and leading to

1

either baccalaureate or master's degrees in nursing). The exit paths enable graduates to sit for the NCLEX-RN licensure exam, and successful passing of this exam means that the individual can practice as a Registered Nurse (RN). There are a wide range of programs and various models for moving from one level of nursing education to another. For example, many schools offer Baccalaureate (BSN) degree programs for applicants who have no previous degrees in nursing (often referred to as accelerated programs for college graduates). These accelerated programs range in length from 12 to 36 months depending on the educational backgrounds of the students. Some schools offer RN completion programs that can range from 1 to 3 years in length depending on the previous educational background of the students. And yet other schools bypass the BSN degree and offer master's level education for either RNs or for college graduates without previous nursing education. As of 2008 there are approximately 1,800 schools of nursing in the United States that offer basic preparation for nurses (eligibility to practice as an RN) (National League for Nursing [NLN], 2008). Between 2005 and 2006, 150 new prelicensure RN programs in nursing were added, and yet the rate of growth in enrollments was only 3% in 2005 and 1.5% in 2006. BSN enrollments grew by only 4.2% in 2006; enrollments in associate degree programs were effectively unchanged, and diploma enrollments fell by 2.6% in 2006 (NLN, 2008).

In 1965, the NLN membership adopted a resolution that supported college-based programs of nursing, calling for the movement of nursing education into institutions of higher education. That same year, 1965, the American Nurses Association (ANA) published its first position statement on nursing education, calling for nursing education within the general system of higher education. The ANA vision was for two levels of nursing education, technical (at the AD level) and professional (at the BSN level) (ANA, 1965).

These early position statements on nursing education at the university level were delivered in the context of broader political discussions of health care. While the position statements were issued almost 20 years after the landmark report of Brown (1948), which called for professional nursing education at the university level, with separate autonomous schools of nursing, the content was similar. Brown contended that the nursing education system was inadequate to meet the nation's health care needs. Until the mid-1960s the professional nursing community did little to implement these changes. But in 1965, the era of the Great Society, there was considerable national debate about health care. Medicare and Medicaid were born, making access to health care available to older persons and the poor. Importantly, at the time of the 1965 position state-ments by both ANA and NLN, approximately 72% of all nurses studied in hospital diploma schools (Donley & Flaherty, 2002). With the societal demand for more nurses and the pressure of hospitals to maintain their supply through hospital-based diploma programs, there was a strong negative reaction to the positions to move nursing to the university level and close diploma programs. To this date, 2008, some diploma programs remain.

Perhaps the most dramatic change since the 1965 position papers has been the rise in associate degree education for RNs. As of 2006, gradu-ates of AD programs represented 41% of all prelicensure RN graduates (NLN, 2008). Graduates of AD, diploma, and BSN pre-licensure pro-grams all are eligible for the same RN licensing examination.

GRADUATE EDUCATION PRIOR TO 1965

In 1952, the NLN held a working conference in Chicago in which criteria for nursing education at the graduate level were developed (Campbell, 1964). One of the key recommendations was that specialty preparation should be at the master's level. According to Fondiller (2001), this confer-ence marked the beginning of a concentrated effort by the NLN Council of Baccalaureate and Higher Degree Programs (CBHDP) to strengthen master's and doctoral education in nursing in clinical specialties, super-vision, administration, teaching, and research (p. 9). Master's degree programs were expanded during the decade following the working con-ference. By 1962 there were 47 master's degree programs in nursing, which enrolled a total of 1,717 full-time students (Campbell, 1964). Many of the early master's degree programs were not clinically focused, but rather offered what were labeled functional minors, in either nurs-ing education or nursing administration. Clinically based master's degree programs grew after the introduction of two forms of clinical specializa-tion, the clinical nurse specialist (CNS) programs and the nurse practi-tioner (NP) programs, both of which were introduced in the mid-1960s.

ADVANCED PRACTICE NURSING EDUCATION

Advanced Practice Nurses (APRNs) include four groups of nurses: clinical nurse specialists (CNSs), nurse anesthetists (CRNAs), nurse midwives (CNMs), and nurse practitioners (NPs). Currently there are about 140,000 APRNs in the United States, including 88,000 NPs, and 54,000 CNSs, the two largest groups of APRNs (Health Resources and Services Administration [HRSA], 2004). There are a wide variety of practice sites for APRNs, including acute and primary care, managed care, and emergency services. Just as there are differences in places of employment, there are a range of employment options, including self-employment, professional practice groups, hospitals and health systems, and managed care organizations. There continues to be some diversity in the scope of practice of APRNs, as this is determined by state, rather than national, legislation. States also set the minimum educational and certification requirements for APRN practice in their jurisdictions. Core competencies for APRN have been described in specialty areas, including those for adult, family, gerontological, pediatric, and women's health NPs. The specialty associations for CRNAs, CNMs, NPs, and CNSs have delineated the competencies for those APRN roles. Presently, all CNSs and NPs are prepared in master's degree or post-master's programs in schools of nursing. The preparation of CRNAs is at the master's degree level as of 1998, and the majority of programs for preparation of CNMs, are at the master's degree level.

All of the APRN roles, have historically had some tensions with organized nursing education, although many of the issues have now been resolved. Initially, there was debate as to whether those practicing as NPs and CRNAs, in particular, were practicing within the scope of nursing or medicine. The practice issues were complicated by the placement of many nurse anesthesia educational programs outside of nursing education, and the placement of NP programs at the certificate level, often under the educational tutelage and, at times, control of both physicians and nurses. CNM practice and education also has had its struggle with nursing, both conceptually and educationally. There has been continued discussion within the American College of Nurse Midwives (ACNM) as to whether midwifery is a separate profession from nursing, even though its origins within nursing are strong.

CRNA Education

The first organized course in anesthesia for graduate nurses was offered in 1909 (American Association of Nurse Anesthetists [AANA], 2008). AANA has its own accrediting commission, which monitors the more than 80 programs that have developed in the past century. Almost half of the programs are in schools of nursing, at the master's degree level. A requirement for master's degree level education as preparation for nurse anesthesia programs has been in effect since 1998. Graduates of CRNA programs are eligible to take the certification exam through the Council on Certification of Nurse Anesthetists (CCNA) (AANA, 2008).

CNM Education

Nurse midwifery education has existed in the United States since 1925 (Varney, Kriebs, & Gegor, 2004). Early in its development, nurse midwifery was viewed as a clinical specialty within nursing (Burst, 2005). The Committee on Organization was formed in 1954; this Committee led to the formation of the ACNM and was organized to set standards for education. ACNM not only accredits nurse-midwifery education programs but also has a component that provides credentialing to nurse-midwives (Burst, 2005). Of the 45 nurse-midwifery programs in place in 2005, 35 are in schools of nursing at the master's degree level. There are four programs in schools of medicine (Burst, 2005).

CNS Education

The first CNS programs in nursing began in the mid-1960s, at the same time that there was much discussion within the profession about the most appropriate degree for entry into professional nursing practice. The primary debate at that time was whether the baccalaureate degree in nursing (BSN) should be required for entry into practice. There also were many societal changes that made health care more available in the United States. The first CNS programs were begun in clinical areas in which there was faculty expertise, such as psychiatric nursing. There also was considerable national funding for development of the specialty of psychiatric nursing in the 1960s. CNSs are prepared as clinical experts in the diagnosis and treatment of illness and the delivery of evidence-based nursing interventions. Presently, there are more than 200 programs preparing CNSs, in a wide range of specialties, including, for example, oncology, cardiovascular, and psychiatric nursing, and specialties that are developmentally focused, such as pediatric and gerontological nursing. The CNS role is focused on the following dimensions: direct clinical practice, expert coaching, collaboration, consultation, research, clinical and professional leadership, and ethical decision making. Historically, the CNS role developed within acute care hospitals but has expanded to other areas (Sparacino, 2005).

NP Education

In 1965, the first NP program was developed at the University of Colorado by Loretta Ford, a nurse, and Henry Silver, a physician. It was a pediatric NP program implemented to meet the need for primary care delivery in underserved areas. Many of the first NP programs were certificate programs, rather than graduate programs. In 1968, Boston College offered one of the first NP programs at the master's degree level, and the University of Colorado program became a master's degree program in the early 1970s (Pulcini & Wagner, 2002). The decade of the 1970s was one in which the number of NP specialties rose, and legislative initiatives were introduced in many states to legitimize the role, particularly within primary care. By 1973 there were over 65 NP programs in the United States; some of these programs granted certificates and some granted master's degrees (Pulcini & Wagner, 2002). The steady growth of NP programs continued for the next 35 years to the present as employment opportunities increased and new NP specialties were introduced. Historically, the NP role began in primary care but has now developed within every component of health care, including acute care hospitals and long-term care facilities.

HISTORY OF DOCTORAL EDUCATION

Doctoral education in nursing began in the first half of the 20th century. The first doctoral degree offered in nursing was in nursing education, offered first at Teachers College, Columbia University in 1933, followed shortly by the EdD offered at New York University (NYU) in 1934 (this program later became the first PhD program in nursing). There was a 20-year hiatus in the opening of new doctoral programs in nursing. The second PhD program in nursing opened in 1954 at the University of Pittsburgh. Then, in the 1960s three Doctor of Nursing Science programs were started, at Boston University (now closed); Catholic University of America in 1968 (now phased into a PhD program as of 2006); and the University of California San Francisco (UCSF) (opened in 1965, closed in the 1990s, but replaced with a PhD program that was opened at UCSF in 1984). The UCSF program was the first doctoral program opened in the West. In early 1970s, there were only seven doctoral programs in nursing: the EdD at Columbia; the PhD programs at NYU, the University of Pittsburgh, and Case Western Reserve University (opened in 1972); and the Doctor of Nursing Science (DNS, also called DNSc) programs at Boston University, Catholic University, and UCSF. The expansion of doctoral programs in nursing occurred in the mid- and late 1970s, with the majority of these opened as PhD programs. There were, however, some universities that would not approve PhD programs in nursing, so the DNS programs, which mimicked PhD programs, were started. By the end of the 1970s there were a total of 17 doctoral programs in nursing (AllNursingSchools Web site; Gortner, 1991; Grace, 1989). The research-oriented doctoral programs in nursing grew more rapidly in the decades of the 1980s and 1990s. By the year 2000 there were 73 research-oriented doctoral programs in nursing (64 PhD and 9 DNS/DNSc/DSN programs) (Fitzpatrick & Stevenson, 2003), and by 2005 there were more than 100 research-oriented doctoral programs (American Association of Colleges of Nursing [AACN], 2005a).

CURRENT STATUS OF GRADUATE PROGRAMS

Master's Degree Programs

Currently there are approximately 400 master's degree programs in nursing, which prepare clinicians, educators, and administrators. According to a report prepared by Walker and colleagues in 2003, there were at least 157 separate CNS programs in 139 schools of nursing (Walker et al., 2003). There are a wide range of CNS specialties, including those that follow the disease status of the recipient of care (oncology or cardiovascular CNS programs) and those that are based on the developmental stage of the recipient of care (pediatric CNS programs). The American Academy of Nurse Practitioners (AANP) identified 850 NP specialty tracks available in over 300 institutions as of 2008 (AANP, 2008). Further noted was the fact that currently only a few NP programs are certificate only, that is, they do not offer any graduate degrees (AANP, 2008). The program tracks for NP preparation include those based on developmental stage, for example, pediatric, adult, geriatric; those based on site of services provision, for example, acute care, emergency room; and those based on groups, for example, family, women (AANP, 2008). The distinctions between CNS and NP programs were historically greater than what currently exists in curricula, with the NP programs more focused on direct care and the CNS programs more focused on indirect care components such as patient and staff education, and consultation with staff. In the recent past, since 2000, there has been a greater emphasis on blended programs (NP plus CNS). Overall, enrollments in master's degree programs rose 18.1% from 2006 to 2007 (AACN, 2007c).

Doctoral Programs

There are approximately 113 research-oriented doctoral programs and 74 practice-oriented doctoral programs. There also are 63 schools of nursing planning clinical doctoral programs at the Doctor of Nursing Practice (DNP) degree level (AACN, 2008a). Research-oriented doctoral programs prepare graduates for careers in academe or in research positions in clinical facilities, whereas the DNP programs prepare graduates for clinical practice positions.

NEW PROGRAMS INTRODUCED BY AACN: THE DOCTOR OF NURSING PRACTICE (DNP) AND THE CLINICAL NURSE LEADER (CNL)

DNP Description

AACN has been deliberating the practice-level doctorate since 2001, which culminated in a vote in support of DNP level education as an entry-level requirement for APRNs by 2015. Formal endorsement of the DNP Position Statement was approved by the AACN membership in 2004 (AACN, 2008b). The AACN "Essentials" document details the history of DNP program development through AACN, essential curricular requirements for DNP graduates, and the plan for future development and implementation (AACN, 2008b).

CNL Description

AACN proposed the CNL as the advanced generalist in nursing (AACN, 2007b). The CNL was conceived as a provider of care for individuals and cohorts, and the role is expected to be implemented across a variety of settings. In its white paper on the CNL, AACN has delineated fundamental aspects of the role, educational requirements, professional values, and core competencies (AACN, 2007b). The CNL is prepared at the master's degree level. The relationship of the CNL (advanced generalist) and CNS (specialist) programs have been delineated in the AACN Working Statement (AACN, 2004).

NUMBER OF NURSES WITH GRADUATE DEGREES

As of 2004, of the total number of registered nurses (N = 2,909,357) living and working in the United States, approximately 376,901 (13%) held a graduate degree (master's or doctorate), according to the national database report (HRSA, 2004). Over the period from 1980 to 2004 there was a 339% increase (from 85,860 to 376,901) in this number (HRSA, 2004). As of 2004, there were 240,460 RNs prepared as Advanced Practice Registered Nurses (APRNs), or 8.3% of the RN population. This estimate represents a 22.5% increase from the estimate in 2000. The majority of those who completed APRN programs were prepared as nurse practitioners (141,209 RNs) followed by CNS-prepared RNs (72,521 RNs). These two groups together account for 82.8% of all APRNs. Nurse anesthetists comprised the third largest group of APRNs, with 32,523 CRNAs in 2004. There were 13,684 nurse midwives (CNMs) as of 2004 (HRSA, 2004).

FACTORS RELATED TO APRN ISSUES

In addition to the changing demographics in the United States, which have increased the overall demand and need for health care, there are other factors directly related to the preparation of APRNs at all levels. These include workforce, education, and practice needs. No one of these dimensions can be addressed independently, and all affect the new educational programs proposed, specifically the DNP and CNL.

Workforce Needs

The current nursing shortage, begun in the middle of this decade, has been identified as the worst ever, with projections varying regarding the numbers of nurses needed by 2020, from 340,000 to earlier projections of 800,000 (AACN, 2007a). Projections of workforce needs are almost always based on the need for basic RNs to fill hospital positions in acute care institutions and do not take into account the needs for APRNs. Yet, it is clear that without the base supply of RNs the enrollment in APRN educational programs will not continue to expand. In times of shortages of RNs, graduate-level enrollments often decline, as nurses have extensive opportunities for employment and often higher levels of compensation. The RN shortage of the current decade has been attributed to the following factors: enrollment in schools of nursing not growing fast enough to meet demand; a shortage of faculty, thus making it impossible to expand programs; the increasing age of the workforce, with projections about large numbers of retirements in the next 10 years; changing demographics, thus increasing the demand for nursing services; job burnout and dissatisfaction and high nurse turnover and vacancy rates (AACN, 2007a).

Education Needs

There is a critical shortage of nurse faculty, one that is predicted to increase as the aging faculty workforce retires. This shortage of faculty is affecting the overall nursing shortage by limiting the number of students who can be accommodated in basic nursing programs. According to the AACN Report on 2007–2008 enrollments, there were 40,285 qualified applicants turned away from baccalaureate and graduate programs primarily due to the faculty shortage (AACN, 2008c). During 2006–2007, AACN reported that 3,306 qualified applicants were turned away from master's degree programs and 299 qualified applicants were turned away from doctoral programs, primarily due to the shortage of faculty (AACN, 2007c). A complicating factor affecting the faculty shortage is that for 307 (78%) of the doctoral graduates who reported their employment plans in the AACN 2004–2005 survey, 22.5% reported that they planned to work in settings other than academe (AACN, 2005b).

Practice Needs

Both NP- and CNS-prepared nurses provide high quality care and make a significant contribution to the overall health care delivery system in a range of practice settings. Outcomes have been linked to safe, high-quality, cost-effective care. Fulton and Baldwin (2004) delineated the outcomes of CNS practice as reduced length of hospital stays, reduced costs, increased patient satisfaction, improved pain management, and fewer complications in hospitalized patients. The positive outcomes of NP practice also have been substantiated (Feldman, Ventura, & Crosby, 1987; Hooker, Cipher, & Skescenski, 2005; Mundinger, Kane, Lenz, Totten, & Tsai, 2002).

SUMMARY

Nursing education has had a complex history, one that has been inextricably linked to the development and delivery of health care services in the United States. There has not been a direct or smooth path in either the educational preparation of APRNs or in the design of the U.S. health care system. The future path also is not clear, and for nursing education and practice, there continue to be several entry and exit points, and a lack of consensus regarding the best road forward.

Currently, there are major issues surrounding nursing education and practice at the advanced levels, including programs to prepare nurses at the DNP and CNL levels. These issues include regulatory and licensure concerns, accreditation of academic programs and credentialing of individual practitioners, and the nature of the educational programs for APRN preparation. AACN has led a 3-year process to develop consensus on these issues and has reported extensively on the developments (AACN, 2007b, 2008b). Each of these issues is complex and will require continued deliberations by key stakeholders in order to chart the future course that is most advantageous to delivery of high-quality nursing and health care.

REFERENCES

AllNursingSchools. Retrieved March 13, 2008, from http://www.allnursingschools.com

American Academy of Nurse Practitioners. (2008). *AANP nurse practitioner program list*. Retrieved March 1, 2008, from http://www.aanp.org

American Association of Colleges of Nursing. (2004). *Working statement comparing the Clinical Nurse Leader and Clinical Nurse Specialist roles: Similarities, differences and complementarities*. Retrieved June 15, 2008, from http://www.aacn.nche.edu

American Association of Colleges of Nursing. (2005a). *Institutions offering doctoral programs in nursing*. Retrieved February 28, 2008, from http://www.aacn.nche.edu

American Association of Colleges of Nursing. (2005b). *Nurse faculty shortage fact sheet*. Retrieved February 28, 2008, from http://www.aacn.nche.edu

American Association of Colleges of Nursing. (2007a). *Nursing shortage fact sheet*. Retrieved February 28, 2008, from http://www.aacn.nche.edu

American Association of Colleges of Nursing. (2007b). *White paper on the education and role of the Clinical Nurse Leader, February, 2007*. Retrieved February 28, 2008, from http://www.aacn.nche.edu

American Association of Colleges of Nursing. (2007c). *American Association of Colleges of Nursing Annual Report 2007*. Retrieved June 15, 2008, from http://www.aacn.nche.edu

American Association of Colleges of Nursing. (2008a). *Doctor of Nursing Practice (DNP) programs*. Retrieved February 28, 2008, from http://www.aacn.nche.edu/DNP/DNPProgramList.htm

American Association of Colleges of Nursing. (2008b). *The essentials of doctoral education for advanced nursing practice*. Retrieved February 28, 2008, from http://www.aacn.nche.edu

American Association of Colleges of Nursing. (2008c). *Nursing faculty shortage fact sheet*. Retrieved June 18, 2008, from http://www.aacn.nche.edu

American Association of Nurse Anesthetists. (2008). *Education of nurse anesthetists in the United States.* Retrieved March 1, 2008, from http://www.aana.org

American Nurses Association. (1965). *A position paper.* New York: Author.

Brown, E. L. (1948). *Nursing for the future.* New York: The Russell Sage Foundation.

Burst, H. V. (2005). The history of nurse-midwifery/midwifery education. *Journal of Midwifery & Women's Health, 50*(2), 129–137.

Campbell, J. (1964). *Masters education in nursing.* New York: National League for Nursing.

Donley, R., & Flaherty, M. J. (2002). Revisiting the American Nurses Association's first position on education for nurses. *OJIN: The Online Journal of Issues in Nursing.* Retrieved 28 February 2008, from http://www.nursingworld.org

Feldman, M. J., Ventura, M. R., & Crosby, F. (1987). Studies of nurse practitioner effectiveness. *Nursing Research, 38,* 303–308.

Fitzpatrick, J. J., & Stevenson, J. S. (2003). A review of the second decade of the *Annual Review of Nursing Research* series. In J. J. Fitzpatrick (Ed.), *Annual Review of Nursing Research* (vol. 21, pp. 335–360). New York: Springer Publishing.

Fondiller, S. H. (2001). The advancement of baccalaureate and graduate nursing education: 1952–1972. *Nursing and Health Care Perspectives, 22*(1), 8–10.

Fulton, J. S., & Baldwin, K. (2004). An annotated bibliography reflecting CNS practice and outcomes. *Clinical Nurse Specialist, 18*(1), 21–39.

Gortner, S. R. (1991). Historical development of doctoral programs: Shaping our expectations. *Journal of Professional Nursing, 7*(1), 45–53.

Grace, H. K. (1989). Issues in doctoral education in nursing. *Journal of Professional Nursing, 7*(1), 45–53.

Health Resources and Services Administration. (2004). *The Registered Nurse population: Findings from the 2004 National Sample Survey of Registered Nurses.* Retrieved August 8, 2008, from http://www.hrsa.gov

Hooker, R. S., Cipher, D. J., & Skescenski, E. (2005). Patient satisfaction with physician assistant, nurse practitioner, and physician care: A national survey of Medicare beneficiaries. *Journal of Clinical Outcomes Management, 12*(2), 88–92.

Mundinger, M. O., Kane, R. L., Lenz, E. R., Totten, A. M., & Tsai, W. (2002). Primary care outcomes in patients treated by nurse practitioners or physicians. *JAMA: Journal of the American Medical Association, 283,* 59–68.

National League for Nursing. (2008). *Nursing data review, academic year 2005–2006.* Retrieved February 29, 2008, from http://www.nln.org

Pulcini, J., & Wagner, M. (2002). Nurse practitioner education in the U.S.: A growing success story. *Clinical Excellence for Nurse Practitioner, 6*(2), 1–6.

Sparacino, P. S. (2005). The clinical nurse specialist. In. A. B. Hamric, J. A. Spross, & C. M. Hanson (Eds.), *Advanced practice nursing: An integrative approach* (3rd ed., pp. 415–446). St. Louis, MO: Elsevier.

Varney, H., Kriebs, J., & Gegor, C. (2004). *Varney's midwifery* (4th ed., pp. 3–27). Sudbury, MA: Jones & Bartlett.

Walker, J., Gerard, P. S., Bayley, E. W., Coeling, H., Clark, A. P., Dayhoff, N., & Goudreau, K. (2003). A description of clinical nurse specialist programs in the United States. *Clinical Nurse Specialist, 17*(1), 50–57. Retrieved February 29, 2008, from http://www.allnursingschools.com

Doctor of Nursing Practice Programs: History and Current Status

2

JOYCE J. FITZPATRICK

In 2004, the American Association of Colleges of Nursing (AACN) membership endorsed the Position Statement on the Practice Doctorate in Nursing (AACN, 2004). This movement toward clinical doctoral education was designed by AACN to address educational program development and practice level needs for Advanced Practice Nurses (APRN). The movement, however, has a history that dates back to the mid-1970s, when there was considerable attention to the development of the discipline of nursing at both conceptual levels and through doctoral program development for PhD education, as well as for clinical and/or professional doctorates. It is important to note that the considerable attention to nursing theory development, and thus, the delineation of the essential content of the discipline of nursing, occurred in the mid-1970s. This national leadership debate about core disciplinary content served as the context in which the first professional doctorate was proposed.

There are several papers in the literature that address the professional, the clinical, and the practice doctorates in nursing. For purposes of this chapter, the terms are used interchangeably. Distinctions are not made as to which author used which term to describe the program under discussion and/or consideration. The program described here is one offered at the post-baccalaureate professional or graduate degree level, labeled either as a professional, practice, or clinical doctorate in nursing.

The organizations that are addressed in this chapter are those that have a critical stake in the future development of graduate programs in nursing. They include the AACN, the National League for Nursing (NLN), the National Organization for Nurse Practitioner Faculties (NONPF), the American Academy of Nurse Practitioners (AANP), the American Association of Nurse Anesthetists (AANA), the American College of Nurse Midwives (ACNM), and the National Association of Clinical Nurse Specialists (NACNS). These four organizations (AANA, AANP, ACNM, and NACNS) have been included, as they are the groups of nurse clinicians who are considered APRNs.

BRIEF HISTORY OF DEVELOPMENT OF CLINICAL DOCTORATES IN NURSING AND DOCTOR OF NURSING PRACTICE (DNP) PROGRAM DEVELOPMENT

In 1979, the first professional doctorate in nursing, the Doctor of Nursing (ND) program was begun at Case Western Reserve University Frances Payne Bolton School of Nursing. Both Christman (1980) and Schlotfeldt (1978) were strong advocates and national leaders in the movement toward professional doctorates in nursing as entry level into practice. One of the key reasons proposed in support of the first professional doctorate at Case was the need to place nursing on a par with educational preparation in other health professions such as medicine and dentistry. There also was the belief that nurses needed a liberal arts and sciences background to deal with the explosion of health care science and clinical knowledge development (Schlotfeldt, 1978).

It is important to note that the widespread development of PhD programs in nursing did not occur until after the first professional doctorate was developed in 1979. The expansion of PhD programs in nursing occurred in the mid-1970s (Gortner, 1991; Grace, 1989). Prior to 1975 there were only three PhD programs in nursing, located at New York University, the University of Pittsburgh, and Case Western Reserve University. From 1975 to 1990 there was a rapid expansion of PhD programs, and a concomitant demand for faculty prepared at the doctoral level to teach in these programs. This societal change was accompanied by the development of research in nursing, including the establishment in 1985 of the National Center for Nursing Research (NCNR) at the National Institutes of Health (NIH). Then in 1993, the NCNR became the National Institute of Nursing Research, a movement that generated support from the entire nursing leadership community and serves as a landmark in nursing collaboration for change.

The initial proposal for the ND program was for entry-level practice in nursing. The leadership model proposed by Schlotfeldt was for replacement of the Baccalaureate of Science in Nursing (BSN) programs at the national level with entry-level professional doctoral programs similar to those in medicine, dentistry, and law. By 1990, due to several factors, including a shortage of nurses that had occurred shortly after the initiation of the ND program, it was apparent that professional doctorate entry-level nursing was not going to occur on a national level. A reassessment of the present ND program occurred at Case, and the decision was made to modify the program so that all graduates were not only prepared for entry-level clinical practice but also were required to be expert practitioners.

In 1990 the Case ND program was changed from an entry-level program to a post-masters clinical doctorate so as to prepare clinicians at the most advanced level of clinical nursing practice (Fitzpatrick, 1989; Fitzpatrick & Modly, 1990). All students enrolled in the program were required to complete a master's degree in nursing to progress to the ND level. Students were eligible to take the NCLEX-RN exam after the first 2 years of the program if they entered without nursing degrees. An active recruitment effort was initiated to enroll nurses with master's degrees in nursing into the ND program, and between 1990 and 2005 several hundred master's-prepared nurses graduated with ND degrees from the Case program. This model of post-master's course work focused on expert nursing practice for APRNs is similar to the current model of Doctor of Nursing Practice (DNP) education developed through AACN and other professional nursing organizations.

AACN ESSENTIALS

AACN describes itself as the national voice for America's baccalaureate and higher-degree nursing education programs. Founded in 1969, partly in reaction to the need to clarify distinctions between levels of nursing education, it is the only national organization devoted exclusively to furthering baccalaureate and graduate-level nursing education. Currently there are more than 600 member institutions that represent large and small public and private colleges and universities.

The AACN history of involvement in developing the practice doctorate has been traced to 2001 at the time of the organization's publication of the third version of the indicators of quality for research-oriented doctoral programs (Lenz, 2005). At that time a task force was formed to explore the issues surrounding relationships between the two types of programs and the potential for introducing a practice doctorate through AACN. From 2004 to 2006 a number of national meetings were held to introduce the potential to the various stakeholders (e.g., schools of nursing with existing graduate programs to prepare APRNs and researchers and APRN professional organization leaders). In 2005, a national stakeholders meeting was held to which 45 professional organizations sent representatives (AACN, 2008b, 2008c).

AACN presented the core content of practice-focused doctoral programs in nursing in a document titled "The Essentials of Doctoral Education for Advanced Nursing Practice" (AACN, 2008c). In this document the historical development of practice-focused degrees in nursing, including the ND degree programs, is detailed. Also included are details regarding the current context of graduate education in nursing, and the key aspects of AACN's proposal for the DNP. The Essential curriculum content for DNP programs includes two domains: foundational competencies and specialty competencies. Foundational competencies are included in the first seven Essentials statements. In the AACN (2008c) document, each of these areas is presented in detail, and student outcomes from each Essential are delineated. The AACN Essentials can be used as guidelines for schools to develop DNP curricula and courses. The Commission on Collegiate Nursing Education (CCNE), which accredits baccalaureate and graduate nursing education programs, has determined that DNP programs must comply with the Essentials in order to be accredited by CCNE (AACN, 2008d). The AACN Essentials as detailed by AACN are as follows:

Essential I: Scientific underpinnings for practice

Core content related to the discipline of nursing, including nursing theories and research, as well as scientific knowledge from other disciplines, is included. Expectations are that students will develop new practice approaches from this knowledge base.

Essential II: Organizational and systems leadership for quality improvement and systems thinking

Core content areas included are related to organizations and policy design and implementation. Students will be expected to develop and evaluate care delivery systems from a variety of perspectives, including organizational, financial, ethical, and quality outcomes.

Essential III: Clinical scholarship and analytical methods for evidence-based practice

Content included is focused on outcome evaluation from the perspective of evidence-based practice, quality improvement models, and the application of information technology and research methods. Students will be expected to be able to apply these various methodologies in their practice.

Essential IV: Information systems/technology and patient care technology for the improvement and transformation of health care

Content included is focused on information systems and technology to support organizational system design, care delivery, and evaluation. Students will be expected to analyze, design, and evaluate information technology and systems as related to their practice and to the health care information needs of clients.

Essential V: Health care policy for advocacy in health care

Content regarding health care policy, including governmental actions, institutional decision making, and organizational standards is included. DNP students are prepared to design, influence and implement health care policy at local, national, and global levels.

Essential VI: Interprofessional collaboration for improving patient and population health outcomes

The content focus is on effective interdisciplinary health care team building and functioning. DNP students will be expected to develop skills in team leadership and collaboration.

Essential VII: Clinical prevention and population health for improving the nation's health

Health promotion, risk reduction, and illness prevention provide the content focus for this Essential. DNP students will develop models of care and care delivery to meet these health goals for various constituents, including individuals, groups, families, and communities.

Essential VIII: Advanced nursing practice

According to the AACN document on the Essentials (2008c), the specialty competencies, content, and practice experiences included in Essential VIII are those delineated by national specialty organizations.

CURRENT PROGRAMS

As of early 2008, according to AACN tracking, there are 74 Doctor of Nursing programs that are operational, with another 63 in the planning stages (AACN, 2008a). The programs are located in very diverse educational institutions, including universities with major academic medical centers, research universities, single-purpose institutions, and small colleges and universities. The programs are located in both public and private colleges and universities.

It is expected that all programs would have the DNP Essentials (AACN, 2007) at the core of the curriculum, there are similarities and differences in the content offered and in the focus for the graduates. The majority of the programs are focused on the preparation of APRNs for expanded advanced practice roles, including leadership, policy development, and informatics. Some of the programs also are focused on the preparation of nurse educators, even though these competencies are outside of the scope of the AACN Essentials. Thus, nurse leaders in executive positions within hospitals are recruited into the DNP programs and provided the knowledge and skills for executive leadership. Nurse leaders in other executive positions, for example, leaders of professional organizations, policy makers, chief nursing officers of health systems, or business owners or managers also are recruited into the DNP programs that emphasize administration and leadership development beyond the Essentials levels. Those who desire positions in nursing education might choose the DNP programs that have curriculum content directly targeted toward preparation of nurse educators. These programs are in the minority, although graduates of DNP programs are actively recruited for faculty positions in newly developed DNP programs. The AACN position is that the DNP's major focus should not be education; rather additional program content should be included in the programs to prepare individuals for the educator role.

There also are differences in the format in which the programs are offered. Some of the programs offer classes only in the traditional face-to-face format in the usual 15-week academic semester, and others offer a blended format of face-to-face and Web-enhanced programming, while still others are totally online programs. Some of the programs incorporate the executive format as the basic program design. These executive models take the form of intensive weekend courses with Web-enhanced experiences, or other versions of condensed immersion programming.

POSITIONS OF KEY ORGANIZATIONS REGARDING THE DNP

NLN Statement

The NLN was begun in 1893 as the American Society of Superintendents of Training Schools for Nurses, the first organization for nursing in the United States. The primary mission of NLN is to promote excellence in nursing education to prepare a strong and diverse nursing workforce. The strategic goals of the organization are directed toward nursing education and nurse educators (NLN, 2008).

The NLN (2007) statement on the DNP addresses the need for preparation of nurse educators with specialized knowledge to engage in the academic enterprise. The concerns regarding the DNP raised by NLN are: (a) DNP graduates may lack the knowledge and skills to fill faculty roles; (b) the programs are not consistent with the need for development of a science of nursing education; (c) there may be a negative impact on the current pool of students engaged in other types of doctoral programs in nursing, particularly problematic at a time of critical shortages of nurse faculty; and (d) there might be a negative impact on funding for research. Further support for the DNP is evident in the NLN statement, particularly in relation to leveling the playing field with other health care professionals and the need for continued DNP program evaluation.

NONPF Position

NONPF began in 1974 and is the only organization specifically devoted to promoting quality nurse practitioner (NP) education at the national and international levels. The mission of NONPF is to provide leadership in promoting quality nurse practitioner education. Through development of instructional skills and scientific investigation in nurse practitioner education, NONPF serves the public interest by assuring the preparation of highly qualified health care professionals (NONPF, 2008).

The NONPF board of directors issued a statement of support regarding the DNP as an important evolutionary step in the preparation of NPs (NONPF, 2006). One key distinction between the NONPF position and the AACN position is that of the deadline that was recommended by AACN, that advanced practice programs should be at the DNP, not the master's degree level, by 2015. NONPF does not support any finite deadline but has encouraged nurse educators in NP programs to make the transition in a smooth manner to maintain the quality of the programs. Further, NONPF supported the need for a national title for practice doctorate programs and endorsed the DNP as the degree title that should be used. The NONPF recommended that the specialty organizations continue to establish and maintain the clinical standards that define the advanced practice role, such as the number of clinical hours required and the requirements for specialty certification. An important contribution of NONPF to the national dialogue regarding DNP programs is the Practice Doctorate Nurse Practitioner Entry-Level Competencies outlined by NONPF (2006), including competencies for independent practice, scientific foundations, leadership, quality, practice inquiry, technology and information literacy, policy health system delivery, and ethics.

AANP Position

AANP was formed in 1985. Its mission is to: promote excellence in NP practice, education, and research; shape the future of health care through advancing health policy; serve as the source of information for NPs, the health care community, and consumers; and build a positive image of the NP role as a leader in the national and global health care community (AANP, 2008).

Along with NONPF, the AANP has been involved in the discussions about the DNP since 2001. An important issue in the national debate, according to AANP (2007) is that the deliberations occur in such a way as to not disenfranchise or denigrate the master's prepared NPs. Key issues raised by AANP include: (a) there should be a commitment to maintain the quality of current programs to prepare NPs who are at master's or post-master's level; (b) there is need for a smooth transition to the new title; (c) curriculum requirements, if any, should be in areas that are recognized to enhance nursing practice; (d) skilled nursing practice should be maintained as the foundation of NP programs; (e) issues related to parity in reimbursement must be addressed; (f) the premature development of programs should be avoided; (g) accreditation standards must be maintained; and (h) programs should remain affordable and accessible in order to maintain an adequate number of NP clinicians (AANP, 2007, pp. 1–2).

AANA Position

AANA was founded in 1931 and is the professional association for more than 36,000 certified registered nurse anesthetists (CRNAs) and student nurse anesthetists. CRNAs are advanced practice nurses who are the providers of 27 million anesthetics given in the United States each year. AANA is the professional association representing CRNAs nationwide. The AANA is dedicated to the professional growth and development of CRNAs by striving to improve the quality of nurse anesthesia education and provide competent providers (AANA, 2008).

The AANA (2006) issued an interim position statement in 2006 expressing lack of support for the AACN position statement and the recommendation that all APRNs must be prepared with DNPs by 2015. AANA has supported the doctoral education as entry into clinical practice for CRNAs to be implemented in 2025 (AANA, 2007).

ACNM Position

ACNM was founded in 1929; its mission is to promote the health and well-being of women and infants within their families and communities through the development and support of the profession of midwifery as practiced by certified nurse-midwives, and certified midwives (ACNM, 2008).

The ACNM position on the DNP is that it is one option for some nurse-midwifery programs but should not be a requirement for entry into midwifery practice (ACNM, 2007). Nurse-midwifery programs are accredited by the ACNM Division of Accreditation.

NACNS Position

Founded in 1995, NACNS exists to enhance and promote the unique, high-value contribution of the clinical nurse specialist to the health and well-being of individuals, families, groups, and communities, and to promote and advance the practice of nursing. Members of NACNS benefit from national, regional, and local efforts of the association to make the contributions of clinical nurse specialists (CNSs) more visible (NACNS, 2008).

NACNS issued a white paper on the DNP in 2005 in which it expressed significant concerns about the DNP as proposed by AACN (NACNS, 2005). The issues raised by NACNS included the need for more CNS-prepared nurses to fill health care needs, replacement of master's-level education with practice doctoral-level education, licensure, regulation, accreditation, and credentialing issues, need for faculty, and concerns about a smooth transition in program implementation.

Current Issues in DNP Education

There are a number of current issues that have been raised in the literature since the active debate was introduced regarding the DNP. These include issues of accreditation, use of the professional title, relationship of the DNP to other doctoral degree programs in nursing, recognition of those currently credentialed as APRNs, interdisciplinary education and practice, the current faculty shortage, and the global context of the movement toward the professional doctorate.

Accreditation

There has not previously been a process in place for accreditation of doctoral programs in nursing. Two bodies presently accredit graduate programs in nursing, the Commission on Collegiate Nursing Education (CCNE) and the National League for Nursing Accrediting Commission (NLNAC). A process for the accreditation of practice doctorates is being designed by CCNE. The specialty organizations for nurse anesthetists and nurse midwives have separate accreditation processes for academic programs. These organizations would necessarily play a role in accreditation of DNP programs that include the tracks for preparation of nurse anesthetists and midwives.

Degree and Professional Titles

According to Pearson (2007) there are currently seven states (Georgia, Illinois, Maine, Missouri, Ohio, Oklahoma, and Oregon) that have statutes or regulations prohibiting an NP from using the title "Doctor." Several states have provisions in law for health professionals to use the title "Doctor" along with their professional title or licensure. The American

Medical Association (AMA) (2006) has opposed the use of the title "Doctor" by NPs and other nonphysician providers and has made this a legislative priority. The AMA position is that the nonphysician providers are misleading patients; the implication is that quality of care will be affected, a position not supported by the research comparing physician and NP providers (Feldman, Ventura, & Crosby, 1987; Hooker, Cipher, & Skescenski, 2005; Mundinger, Kane, Lenz, Totten, & Tsai, 2002).

As all professionals, DNP-prepared nurses must be cognizant of the state regulations and laws regarding their clinical practice and their title recognition. Importantly as well, given the fluidity of the development of DNP education and the degree recognition at state levels, DNP-prepared nurses should become involved at the policy and public levels to create opportunities for enhancing quality patient care and nursing education.

Recognition of Current Credentials of APRNs

One debate among practicing APRNs is whether or not those who are nationally certified should have to complete additional education to qualify for the DNP credential. The issue is one of "grandfathering" (or "grandmothering" as often used in nursing), these individuals into the new status. While the preparation for clinical credentialing is one aspect of DNP education, there are other dimensions of the educational programs that are post-master's content. Thus, it is highly unlikely that any universities would automatically confer the DNP degree on previous graduates of Master's Degree in Nursing (MSN) advanced practice programs. In the case of individual programs in which the degree granted was an ND in which course work was offered at a post-master's doctoral level, individual graduates can request authority from the university to use the new degree and professional credential.

Nursing has a long history of changes in program requirements for different levels of preparation, and an equally long history of confusion (and diversity) in recognition of previous academic preparation. For example, the progression to baccalaureate-level education for individuals who entered nursing through associate degree and diploma-level programs has not always been smooth. Originally many nurses were required to enter as new students, with none of their previous nursing education recognized. Presently there is often blanket recognition of the previous education if the student has the Registered Nurse (RN) credential. BSN degree completion programs provide add-on material only, thus facilitating the student progression to BSN level. This transition took several years, though, and it is likely that there will be substantive and continued discussions regarding the content of DNP programs that requires the APRN to enroll in post-master's courses. Most of the current DNP programs are specifically designed to accommodate those APRNs who desire the post-master's content. Yet the core content required ranges across programs from approximately 25 academic credits to more than 75 academic credits. In addition, some of the programs require additional clinical credits and supervised experiences, similar to residency programs, while others concentrate on the leadership, health policy, research- and evidence-based practice, and informatics dimensions in program development. If the nursing education community moves toward accreditation of the DNP programs, there may be more standardization of content. But presently the diversity of requirements is confusing for students and faculty, as well as the public.

Relationships to Other Degrees in Nursing

There are other types of doctoral degrees offered in nursing, including the Doctor of Philosophy (PhD), the Doctor of Education (EdD), and the Doctor of Nursing Science (DNS or DNSc) and Doctor of Science in Nursing (DSN). Minnick and Halstead (2002) surveyed the 87 doctoral programs in nursing in existence at the time. This included 71 PhD programs, 7 DNSc programs, and 4 DNS/DSN programs. At that time there also were four ND programs, all of which have now converted their degrees and programs to DNP degrees. As of 2004 there were 96 doctoral programs in nursing in the United States, with the majority (76) PhD programs and 13 DNS/DNSc programs (Pastor, Cimiotti, & Stone, 2004). Some of the Doctor of Nursing Science programs have recently been converted to PhD programs in nursing. While there are 113 research-based doctoral programs in nursing, there is no evidence that the DNP programs are diluting the focus of these programs.

The research-based and practice-based doctoral programs serve different purposes in the discipline of nursing. Nurses are needed for expert clinical knowledge generation and for scientific research; clinical and research ways of knowing are different in a clinical discipline such as nursing and require different skill sets (Fitzpatrick, 2002). The history of doctoral programs in nursing, including both the PhD and the DNS/DSN/DNSc programs is detailed in the literature (Anderson, 2000; Gortner, 1991; Robb, 2005). None of the other degree programs resemble the proposed DNP programs or the DNP programs currently operating. While the Doctor of Nursing Science degree programs were originally construed to be practice oriented (Downs, 1989), they quickly drifted into research-oriented programs and often mimicked PhD programs. Thus, the PhD and DNS/DSN/DNSc programs are similar to each other and are research-based programs. They include philosophy and theories of nursing, and research methods and content (Wood, 2005). The EdD programs are focused on preparation of nurses for nursing research in nursing education and the preparation of nurse faculty.

Some nurse academics have argued that the introduction of the new DNP degree will detract from the current programs (Dracup, Cronenwett, Meleis, & Benner, 2005; Meleis & Dracup, 2005) in terms of time and energy spent in the deliberations and program design. The degree distinction, the basic content, however, should be the key factor that supports new program development, rather than the sociological or psychological arguments proposed by Meleis and Dracup. There is no evidence that the DNP programs will detract from the PhD programs in nursing. The argument can be proposed that the DNP programs will help to strengthen PhD programs (Fitzpatrick, 2003), as many of the PhD programs are not strong research programs. Rather, students have been attracted to PhD programs in nursing as there were no other alternatives for doctorates in nursing. Many students currently enrolled in PhD programs are not committed to careers as nurse scientists. Thus, it can be argued that it is a waste of resources to prepare nurses at the PhD level who will not pursue research careers, either in the traditional academic setting as faculty or in clinical research roles within health care environments (Fitzpatrick, 2003).

Another concern that is apparent within the academic circles and has also been raised in the literature is that the DNP will become a second-class degree and the graduates will be treated as second-class citizens within the academic community (Meleis & Dracup, 2005). Again, one has only to look to medicine in order to structure the future environment for academic nursing. DNP graduates should be afforded the highest respect as expert clinicians, with the power, authority, and responsibility for advancing the care of patients in concert with professional colleagues in health care. They should have the authority over clinical education programs, much as expert APRNs are currently responsible for the design and monitoring of current programs to meet credentialing and accreditation requirements. At the same time, within major academic research institutions, often driven by the scientific processes of research and publication, the PhD will always be accorded the highest academic stature. Thus, it is unfair to make the comparison between the DNP and the PhD on academic credentials alone. The skill sets required for each are different, as are the ways of knowing and being (Fitzpatrick, 2002). Thus, the core of the DNP graduate work should be expert clinical practice and education, and the core of the PhD graduate work should be research and the scholarship of education.

RENEWED RECOGNITION FOR EMPHASIS ON INTERDISCIPLINARY EDUCATION AND PRACTICE

As noted by the Institute of Medicine (2003), the current and future need is for health professionals prepared together through interdisciplinary education to engage in collaborative interprofessional practice. This recommendation is not new and has its roots in the development of models of primary health care. The DNP program development will position nursing and nurses to be equal members of the interdisciplinary team. With the education of APRNs on the same level as other team members, there are enhanced opportunities for collaboration in practice. There is substantial research evidence that collaboration and team functioning among health professionals leads to better-quality care (Shaver, 2005).

The Severe Faculty Shortage

The shortage of doctorally prepared nurse faculty has been documented in the literature, with predictions that without direct attention to short- and long-term solutions, the shortage will not be resolved (Berlin & Sechrist, 2002). Yet, it has been argued that the preparation of more DNP-prepared nurses will ease the current severe faculty shortage (Fitzpatrick, 2003). In a professional practice discipline the need is for expert clinicians, not researchers, to teach basic and advanced clinical-practice students. Those with DNP degrees will be prepared to assume these roles; just as in other health science disciplines, the clinical content is taught by clinicians and the clinical supervision is by experts in direct clinical practice. The DNP degree will qualify individuals for appointments at professorial rank and full membership in the academic community, which requires an earned doctorate. Thus far, within the boundaries of academe, nursing has often been the exception to the rule, as many nurse faculty members now have only the master's degree as their highest credential. The DNP degree will place nurse clinicians who assume faculty positions on a par with physicians and dentists who are in faculty positions. Appointments for physicians with MD degrees and dentists with DDS degrees can be made at the level of assistant professor and above as the MD and DDS degrees are considered earned doctorates. Often, nurse faculty members with master's degrees are restricted within the academic environment. Most often, without the earned doctorate, nurse faculty members assume appointments as instructors or lecturers.

Global Context

Doctoral education in nursing is developing throughout the world, as is the debate about the types of doctoral preparation that are most suited for the discipline. Even within the PhD degree programs, significant differences exist in the models that are in place in different countries (Wood, 2005). At the same time, there are discussions about the differences and similarities and the needs and requirements for the professional and research doctorates in nursing in other countries as well as the United States (Ellis, 2005, 2006, 2007). This debate is likely to be accelerated as the DNP becomes more common in the United States and the preparation of APRNs is expanded in other countries.

SUMMARY

While the dialogue regarding the DNP has been strong at the nursing education and advanced practice levels, there is a current need to engage all nurse leaders in the discussion (Fulton & Lyon, 2005; Glazer, 2005). We have been reminded that the question is no longer whether the DNP is "future or fringe" as it was originally characterized (Marion et al., 2003), but rather how to shape the future of DNP programs (O'Sullivan, Carter, Marion, Pohl, & Werner, 2005).

But importantly, for the movement to be successfully implemented, there also needs to be attention at levels of state policy, including financial planning to support programs in public institutions of higher education, and deliberations by state regulatory agencies that set requirements for advanced practice title recognition. Cartwright and Reed (2005) proposed a proactive change process for DNP implementation, outlining key elements at the external public policy level and internal to the nursing education and practice communities. One of the key elements identified is that of resources necessary to implement the changes, including financial and personnel resources (Cartwright & Reed, 2005). The 10-year transition plan allows for managed change but has not been uniformly accepted by key professional organizations such as NONPF and AANP. Without careful attention to all of the key dimensions of the planned change for replacement of master's-level APRN education with DNP-level education, the road to the DNP may be fraught with similar challenges as the entry into practice issue in nursing education.

REFERENCES

American Academy of Nurse Practitioners. (2007). *Discussion paper: Doctor of Nursing Practice.* Washington, DC: Author.

American Academy of Nurse Practitioners. (2008). Retrieved February 29, 2008, from http://www.aanp.org

American Association of Colleges of Nursing. (2004). *AACN position statement on the practice doctorate in nursing.* Retrieved May 30, 2008, from http://www.aacn.nche.edu/DNP/pdf/DNP.pdf

American Association of Colleges of Nursing. (2008a). *Doctor of Nursing Practice (DNP) programs.* Retrieved February 28, 2008, from http://www.aacn.nche.edu/DNP/DNP ProgramList.htm

American Association of Colleges of Nursing. (2008b). *Doctor of Nursing Practice (DNP) programs: Frequently asked questions. Last updated February 11, 2008.* Retrieved February 28, 2008, from http://www.aacn.nche.edu

American Association of Colleges of Nursing. (2008c). The essentials of doctoral education for advanced nursing practice. Retrieved February 28, 2008, from http://www.aacn.nche.edu

American Association of Colleges of Nursing. (2008d). *Frequently asked questions DNP programs and CCNE accreditation.* Retrieved June 18, 2008, from http://www.aacn.nche.edu

American Association of Nurse Anesthetists. (2006). *Interim position statement on the DNP as entry into advanced practice for nurse anesthetists: February, 2006.* Retrieved February 28, 2008, from http://www.aana.com

American Association of Nurse Anesthetists. (2007). *AANA position statement on doctoral preparation of nurse anesthetists: Adopted June 2, 2007.* Retrieved June 15, 2008, from http://www.aana.com

American Association of Nurse Anesthetists. (2008). Retrieved February 28, 2008, from http://www.aana.com

American College of Nurse-Midwives. (2007). *Position statement: Midwifery education and the Doctor of Nursing Practice (DNP).* Retrieved February 28, 2008, from http://www.acnm.org

American College of Nurse-Midwives. (2008). Retrieved February 28, 2008, from http://www.acnm.org

American Medical Association. (2006). *House of Delegates Resolution 211 (A-06), June 13, 2006.* Retrieved October 22, 2007, from http://www.ama-assn.org/ama1/pub/upload/mm/471/211a06.doc

Anderson, C. E. (2000). Current strengths and limitations of doctoral education in nursing: Are we prepared for the future? *Journal of Professional Nursing, 16*(4), 1919–2000.

Berlin, L. E., & Sechrist, K. R. (2002). The shortage of doctorally prepared nursing faculty: A dire situation. *Nursing Outlook, 50*(2), 50–56.

Cartwright, C. A., & Reed, C. K. (2005). Policy and planning perspectives for the doctorate in nursing practice: An educational perspective. *Online Journal of Issues in Nursing, 10*(3). Retrieved October 14, 2005, from http://www.nursingworld.org/ojin/topic28/tpc28_6.htm

Christman, L. (1980). Leadership in practice. *Image: Journal of Nursing Scholarship, 12*, 31–33.

Downs, F. A. (1989). Differences between the professional doctorate and the academic/research doctorate. *Journal of Professional Nursing, 5*(5), 261–265.

Dracup, K., Cronenwett, L., Meleis, A. I., & Benner, P. E. (2005). Reflections on the doctorate of nursing practice. *Nursing Outlook, 53*(4), 177–182.

Ellis, L. (2005). Professional doctorates for nurses: Mapping provision and perceptions. *Journal of Advanced Nursing, 50*, 440–448.

Ellis, L. (2006). The professional doctorate for nurses in Australia: Findings of a scoping exercise. *Nurse Education Today, 26*, 484–493.

Ellis, L. (2007). Academics' perceptions of the professional or clinical doctorate: Findings of a national survey. *Journal of Clinical Nursing, 16*(12), 2272–2277.

Feldman, M. J., Ventura, M. R., & Crosby, F. (1987). Studies of nurse practitioner effectiveness. *Nursing Research, 38*, 303–308.

Fitzpatrick, J. J. (1989). The professional doctorate as an entry level into professional practice. In *Perspectives in nursing, 1987–1989* (pp. 53–56). New York: National League for Nursing.

Fitzpatrick, J. J. (2002). The balance in nursing: Clinical and scientific ways of knowing and being. *Nursing Education Perspectives, 23*(2), 57.

Fitzpatrick, J. J. (2003). *The case for the clinical doctorate in nursing. Reflections on nursing leadership.* Indianapolis, IN: Sigma Theta Tau International.

Fitzpatrick, J. J., & Modly, D. M. (1990). The first Doctor of Nursing (ND) program. In N. L. Chasta (Ed.), *The nursing profession: Tuning points.* St. Louis, MO: Mosby.

Fulton, J. S., & Lyon, B. L. (2005). The need for some sense making: Doctor of nursing practice. *Online Journal of Issues in Nursing, 10*(3). Retrieved October 14, 2005, from http://www.nursingworld.org/ojin/topic28/tpc28_3.htm

Glazer, G. (2005). Overview and summary: The Doctor of Nursing Practice (DNP): Need for more dialogue. *Online Journal of Issues in Nursing, 10*(3). Retrieved October 14, 2005, from http://www.nursingworld.org/ojin/topic28/tpc28ntr.htm

Gortner, S. R. (1991). Historical development of doctoral programs: Shaping our expectations. *Journal of Professional Nursing, 7*(1), 45–53.

Grace, H. K. (1989). Issues in doctoral education in nursing. *Journal of Professional Nursing, 7*(1), 45–53.

Hooker, R. S., Cipher, D. J., & Skescenski, E. (2005). Patient satisfaction with physician assistant, nurse practitioner, and physician care: A national survey of Medicare beneficiaries. *Journal of Clinical Outcomes Management, 12*(2), 88–92.

Institute of Medicine. (2003). *Health professions education: A bridge to quality.* Washington, DC: National Academies Press.

Lenz, E. R. (2005). The practice doctorate in nursing: An idea whose time has come. *Online Journal of Issues in Nursing, 10*(3). Retrieved October 14, 2005, from http://www.nursingworld.org/ojin/topic28/tpc28_1.htm

Marion, L. N., Viens, D., O'Sullivan, A. L., Crabtree, K., Fontana, S., & Price, M. M. (2003). The practice doctorate in nursing: Future or fringe? *Topics in Advanced Practice Nursing E-Journal, 3*(2). Retrieved May 30, 2008, from http://www.medscape.com/viewarticle/500742

Meleis, A. I., & Dracup, K. (2005). The case against the DNP: History, timing, substance, and marginalization. *Online Journal of Issues in Nursing, 10*(3). Retrieved October 14, 2005, from http://www.nursingworld.org/ojin/topic28/tpc28_2.htm

Minnick, A. F., & Halstead, J. A. (2002). A data-based agenda for doctoral education reform. *Nursing Outlook, 50*(1), 24–29.

Mundinger, M. O., Kane, R. L., Lenz, E. R., Totten, A. M., & Tsai, W. (2002). Primary care outcomes in patients treated by nurse practitioners or physicians. *JAMA: Journal of the American Medical Association, 283,* 59–68.

National Association of Clinical Nurse Specialists. (2005). *White paper on the nursing practice doctorate: April 2005.* Retrieved March 1, 2008, from http://www.nacns.org

National Association of Clinical Nurse Specialists. (2008). Retrieved March 1, 2008, from http://www.nacns.org

National League for Nursing. (2007). *Reflection and dialogue: Doctor of Nursing Practice (DNP).* Retrieved February 29, 2008, from http://www.nln.org

National League for Nursing. (2008). *Mission and goals.* Retrieved February 29, 2008, from http://www.nln.org

National Organization of Nurse Practitioner Faculties. (2006). *Statement on the practice doctorate in nursing: Response to recommendations on clinical hours and degree title.* Retrieved February 28, 2008, from http://www.nonpf.com/NONPF/PracticeDoctorateResourceCenter

National Organization of Nurse Practitioner Faculties. (2008). Retrieved February 28, 2008, from http://www.nonpf.com

O'Sullivan, A. L., Carter, M., Marion, L., Pohl, J. M., & Werner, K. E. (2005). Moving forward together: The practice doctorate in nursing. *Online Journal of Issues in Nursing, 10*(3). Retrieved October 14, 2005, from http://www.nursingworld.org/ojin/topic28/tpc28_4.htm

Pastor, D. K., Cimiotti, J. P., & Stone, P. W. (2004). Doctoral preparation in nursing: What are the options? *Applied Nursing Research, 17*(2), 137–139.

Pearson, L. (2007). The Pearson report. *American Journal of Nurse Practitioners, 11,* 2.

Robb, W. J. (2005). PhD, DNSc, ND: The ABCs of nursing doctoral degrees. *Dimensions of Critical Care Nursing, 24*(2), 86–96.

Scholtfeldt, R. M. (1978). The professional doctorate: Rationale and characteristics. *Nursing Outlook, 26,* 302–311.

Shaver, J. L. (2005). Interdisciplinary education and practice: Moving from reformation to transformation. *Nursing Outlook, 53*(2), 57–58.

Wood, M. J. (2005). Comparison of doctoral programs: The United States, the United Kingdom, and Canada. *Clinical Nursing Research, 14*(1), 3–10.

The Doctor of Nursing Practice: Historical Trends, Major Issues, and Theoretical Underpinnings

3

LINDA THOMPSON ADAMS, KERRI SCHUILING, AND FRANCES JACKSON

Health care in the United States is a major concern for business and civic leaders, policy makers, and consumers because of rising costs, mounting quality problems, and increasing numbers of citizens without health insurance (Adams & O'Neil, 2008). The Pew Health Professions Commission (Finocchio et al., 1995) argued for the redesign of health professional education to address the increasing complexity of the health care system. Further, the Institute of Medicine (IOM) report called for new directions in, and emphasis on, the education of health care professionals to achieve core competencies in patient-centered care, integration of an interdisciplinary approach to health care management, use of evidence-based practice, continuous quality improvement, and the incorporation of informatics to manage and understand the wealth of data available to clinicians (IOM, 2003). One strategy proposed by nurse leaders was to accept the practice doctorate as the terminal degree of an advanced practice nurse (AACN, 2004). This chapter includes a presentation of historical trends of the practice doctorate in nursing, major issues in implementation, and theoretical considerations.

Recently, interest in the practice doctorate in nursing has increased because of several trends in nursing and health professional education, including the increasing complexity of health care resulting in the need for additional knowledge for practice, the trend toward practice doctorates as entry to practice, the increase in credit requirements at the master's level in nursing, and the need for nursing-prepared faculty for clinical teaching.

Schlotfeldt (1978) and other nurse leaders (Fitzpatrick, 1989; Grace, 1989) originally conceptualized the nursing doctorate (ND) as an entry-level practice degree. Although the early ND degree programs failed to be embraced by the nursing community, their development contributed to the discipline by offering a practice-focused doctoral degree that was purposively different from the research-focused doctorates, for example, PhD, Doctor of Nursing Science (DNS or DNSc), and Doctor of Science in Nursing (DSN) (Lenz, 2005). Today, some would say the leaders who originally proposed the idea for a practice doctorate were ahead of their time, if not exceptionally visionary.

Currently, there is a resurgence of practice-focused doctoral degree programs, which, in large part, is attributable to the American Association of Colleges of Nursing's (AACN) *Position Statement on the Practice Doctorate in Nursing* (2004) and the continued ongoing work of the AACN and National Organization of Nurse Practitioner Faculties (NONPF). Both organizations encourage the professoriate to adopt the Doctor of Nursing Practice (DNP) as the terminal practice degree for advanced practice nurses (APRNs).

The idea that the two types of programs are distinctly different and should not be evaluated by identical criteria is consistent with the recommendations of a task force of the AACN that reviewed and recommended the indicators of quality for research-focused nursing doctoral programs (AACN, 2001). During this time, the idea that the nursing discipline should offer both research- and practice-focused doctoral degrees had resurfaced and was beginning to stimulate considerable discussion and activity. Three additional schools of nursing were then planning, and later opened, practice-focused doctoral programs: the University of Tennessee Health Science Center, the University of Kentucky, and Columbia University.

REVIEW OF MAJOR ISSUES

Concerns about the DNP fall into one or more of the following three broad categories: (a) education, (b) economics, and (c) practice. This section identifies some of the more salient issues within these categories and reviews them from historical, societal, economic, and contemporary practice perspectives.

The AACN position statement, in addition to several recommendations, identifies a deadline of 2015, by which all advanced nursing practice programs should be at the DNP level (AACN, 2004). The 2015 deadline is a significant issue for a number of advanced practice nursing programs, because many are not located in institutions that have the authority or accreditation status to offer a doctoral degree (O'Sullivan, Carter, Marion, Pohl, & Werner, 2005). The move to offering a DNP degree would require these universities to either receive approval to grant doctoral degrees or authorize an affiliation agreement between a current doctoral degree-granting institution and an institution without authority or accreditation looking to implement the DNP program (O'Sullivan, 2005). In some states this process is lengthy and will require additional use of scarce resources. In many states, collaborating with another university can be costly and may negatively impact the receipt of public funds, especially if those funds are based on numbers of graduates.

The economic impact on educational resources and costs to students are also concerns. Proponents of the DNP argue convincingly that advanced practice nursing programs are already credit-heavy, and the degree awarded, the master's, is not commensurate with the number of credits currently required for the degree. A number of university master's degree programs range from 30–40 credit hours; however, many nursing master's programs require 45 to 50 credit hours (and some even more) (Hathaway, Jacob, Stegbauer, Thompson, & Graff, 2006). Additionally, the required number of clinical hours for APRN students has increased over the years (Hathaway et al., 2006), which creates an inequity in the degrees awarded by an institution (Brown et al., 2006). Thus, it appears student costs and the amount of time it will take to earn a DNP may not increase significantly, and the benefit is that the student receives a degree more in line with the number of credits earned.

The cost of accrediting DNP programs raises yet another economic issue. Professional organizations such as the National League for Nursing Accrediting Commission (NLNAC) and the Commission on Collegiate Nursing Education (CCNE) will offer accreditation for DNP programs. Although not required, accreditation significantly benefits programs that are accredited in many ways. The cost of accreditation is significant and the process time-consuming. Thus, accreditation will add a financial burden to universities offering the DNP.

Many in the professoriate question whether or not DNP programs will create a drain on admissions to research-focused doctoral programs. Those opposed to the DNP argue that the programs will negatively impact research-focused programs because the two programs will compete with one another for applicants (Fulton & Lyon, 2005).

O'Sullivan and colleagues (2005) and Hathaway and colleagues (2006) suggest the contrary and believe DNP programs benefit research-focused programs. Hathaway and colleagues observed that existing DNP programs, within universities that also offer a PhD, positively impact PhD programs, because the situation provides opportunity for discussion about doctoral education, and those discussions aid in the recruitment for more students to doctoral programs, both DNP and PhD. O'Sullivan and colleagues suggest the DNP will help to preserve the integrity of PhD programs as the true research degree, because there is now a choice for nurses who are practice-focused and do not want to develop programs of research, but who desire to expand their practice knowledge about leadership, policy, organizations, systems, informatics, and evidence-based research that includes the use of evidence to improve practice (Bartels, 2005).

Nursing education and practice responds to societal needs for health care. As societal needs for health care grew and nursing care increased in complexity, nursing education moved from hospital-based diploma programs to university-based programs that provide curricula undergirded by a scientific foundation. As the advanced practice role continues to evolve, it requires clinicians to have more knowledge and higher-level skills. This comes at a cost to both employers of DNPs and to consumers of health care. As the depth of education increases, there tends to be a concomitant increase in the salaries of clinicians (Dracup, Cronenwett, Meleis, & Benner, 2005). It is not yet known if the benefit of a DNP education will offset the cost. Also, the contribution to health care systems of those prepared at the DNP level is not yet established (Otterness, 2006).

Practice is emphasized throughout DNP curricula and embedded in all didactic courses (Hathaway et al., 2006). The new degree and title will require educating the public about APRN education, a public that is already confused by the many educational routes and titles used in nursing and health care in general. Uniform credentialing, titling, and licensure will help to alleviate some of this confusion. Ultimately, it is the role of individual professionals and not the professionals' degrees that make the difference to patients (Hathaway, et al., 2006).

There remain many unknowns about the impact of the DNP. Foremost is the question of how this advanced degree will affect the outcomes of patient care. Proponents believe that clinicians who earn DNPs are the experts in clinical practice. They will evaluate current practices and develop evidence-based guidelines for patient care. These nurses prepared at the practice doctorate level will effectively reduce the practice theory gap (Yam, 2005).

It is imperative that the profession of nursing begin in earnest now to track the outcomes of DNP programs and DNP providers as well as patients who are the recipients of their care. Quality assurance and continuous program evaluation are critical to evaluating the effectiveness of the degree and to maintaining quality within the programs offering the degree.

THEORETICAL AND RESEARCH PERSPECTIVES

The establishment of the DNP as a terminal practice degree in nursing is an exciting development that opens endless possibilities for the nursing profession. It generates many questions by nurses and non-nurses. A key issue is the comparison of the DNP to the PhD. How are they the same? How are they different? Is there some overlap? From discussions at national meetings it appears that most questions focus on the theoretical and research content in the DNP curriculum. The DNP Essentials provide a guide for specific content about theory and research that should be included in the DNP curriculum.

Theoretical Perspective

Essential I: Scientific Underpinning for Practice identifies the need for DNP curricula to use science-based theories as a foundation for practice (AACN, 2004). At the Master of Science in Nursing (MSN) level, students are introduced to the scientific underpinnings of practice, which includes a strong emphasis on nursing theories that are the foundation of practice. This foundation provides the framework for a number of middle-range theories that can guide nursing practice.

The Essentials of Doctoral Education for Nursing Practice (AACN, 2006) state the practice doctorate will have less emphasis on theory and meta-theory (AACN, 2004, p. 3). However, in our recent experience with DNP students, we found that it was not less emphasis that was needed, but rather a broader inclusion of a number of middle-range theories that would not only support clinical practice, but that might also be useful for collaborative research. Such theories/conceptual models as the theory of reasoned action, social cognitive theory, change theory, the transtheoretical model, the health belief model, and others can provide the conceptual foundation for clinical interventions and add to the support for evidence-based practice. Interventions that are theoretically based are more amenable to testing and replication. The importance of this foundation cannot be overstated. In the first class of 20 DNP graduates in the joint DNP program at Northern Michigan University and Oakland University in Rochester, Michigan, almost all students used a middle-range theory from nursing or related health sciences as the basis for their evidence-based practice interventions. Since the interventions implemented were consistent with the conceptual model, this supported the idea that the exposure of the DNP student to a broad array of middle-range theories was warranted.

Students who have non-nursing master's degrees and who lack the introductory course work in nursing theory struggled with the advanced theory course and had difficulty making the connection between conceptual models and clinical practice. With the focus on evidence-based practice and translational research that is a distinguishing feature of the DNP graduate, the foundation in nursing theory and middle-range theories is a critical part of DNP education and is part of the "bridge" that the DNP graduate will span between the staff nurse and the PhD research scholar (Magyary, Whitney, & Brown, 2006). Given that one of the goals of the DNP Essentials is to prepare graduates who can "develop and evaluate new practice approaches based on nursing theories and theories from other disciplines," the focus on nursing and middle-range theories is supported and warranted.

The PhD-prepared scholar will certainly have some of the same theoretical foundations. Beyond advanced nursing theory or meta-theory, it is possible the PhD nurse scholar may be well acquainted with the conceptual models that drive and support a particular line of research. It is possible the DNP graduate will not have the depth of theoretical knowledge of the PhD-prepared scholar but instead have a broader range of knowledge of middle-range theories that support evidence-based practice. As the role of the DNP graduate continues to evolve, the level and type of theoretical or conceptual knowledge needed for the expected role of this practitioner will also evolve and be refined and focused.

Research

The graduate of a DNP program is expected to play a major role in translational research, with the ultimate goal that he or she will transform and improve health care. This practitioner will help to bridge the gap between the theoretical foundations for clinical practice, and the implementation or operationalization of models in clinical practice (Magyary, Whitney, & Brown, 2006). Both the PhD and the DNP curricula have scholarly expectations; however, the DNP curriculum places less emphasis on research methodology and statistics than in typical PhD curricula (or programs). DNP graduates need sufficient research to implement and evaluate health care practices and outcomes. They are also expected to participate in collaborative research (AACN, 2004).

The focus for the DNP graduate is on quality improvement, including the ability to apply research and to carry out the design, implementation, and evaluation of research. Emphasis is placed on the critical appraisal of evidence, as well as critical appraisal of strengths and limitations of diverse methodologies, used to generate evidence to promote safe, timely, effective, efficient, and equitable patient-centered health care.

DNP graduates are not given the research skills to generate new knowledge or to conduct meta-analyses; however, they do need sufficient background to critically appraise research and to evaluate outcomes. The following course objectives are taken from our advanced research course for DNP students (Oakland University School of Nursing, 2006):

NRS 890 Course Objectives

1   Use research and continuous quality improvement methods to collect relevant and accurate data to generate evidence for nursing practice.
2   Use research and continuous quality improvement methods to design, direct, and evaluate research and quality improvement initiatives.
3   Use analytic methods to critically evaluate existing literature and other evidence to determine and implement practice initiatives based on best evidence.
4   Analyze strengths and weaknesses of population-based and hospital based case-control studies and related studies as a basis for implementing evidence-based practice initiatives.
5   Evaluate the value of diverse research designs for controlling the confounding effects of extraneous variables on research and continuous quality improvement initiatives.

After this course was taught for the first time, it was recognized that additional content was needed on qualitative research. However, the objectives remained the same.

The clinical role of the DNP graduate is expected to expand, become more collaborative, and broaden to encompass the health care of populations and system-wide care. The focus of the DNP is not to increase clinical expertise per se; rather the goal is provide the foundation for increased clinical leadership. The DNP degree graduate will serve as a "bridge" between the PhD-prepared nurse scholar and the staff nurse, helping to promote and implement translational research. In this regard, the additional foundation in theory and research is a crucial part of the DNP curriculum.

SUMMARY AND FUTURE DIRECTIONS

In this chapter the practice and educational trends that led to the resurgence of interest in the practice doctorate in nursing were reviewed. The characteristics of existing practice doctoral programs and differences between practice and research-focused programs were explicated. Potential benefits of the degree for health care and for nursing education were detailed. Several of the issues that were taken into account in the development of the AACN position paper on the practice doctorate were described. These included the scope of the degree, the recommendations regarding a core curricular structure and content areas for inclusion, and the controversial decision to recommend that the DNP be established as the terminal degree for advanced nursing practice.

As we look ahead, many issues remain to be resolved and many challenges remain to be addressed. There is considerable work to be done by individuals and groups in practice, educational, and regulatory arenas. However, if excitement, interest, and the number of institutions moving forward to develop DNP programs are valid indicators, then the practice-focused doctorate in nursing is an idea whose time has come.

REFERENCES

Adams, L. T., & O'Neil, E. H. (2008). *The nurse executive: The four principles of management.* New York: Springer Publishing.

American Association of Colleges of Nursing. (2001). *Indicators of quality in research-focused doctoral programs in nursing.* Retrieved June 12, 2008, from http://www.aacn.nche.edu

American Association of Colleges of Nursing. (2004). *AACN position statement on the practice doctorate in nursing.* Retrieved February 9, 2008, from http://www.aacn.nche.edu/DNP/DNPPositionStatement.htm

American Association of Colleges of Nursing. (2006). *The essentials of doctoral education for advanced nursing practice.* Retrieved May 15, 2008, from http://www.aacn.nche.edu

Bartels, J. (2005). Educating nurses for the 21st century. *Nursing and Health Sciences, 7,* 221–225.

Brown, M. A., Draye, M. A., Zimmer, P. A., Magyary, D., Woods, S., Whitney, J., et al. (2006). Developing a practice doctorate in nursing: University of Washington perspectives and experience. *Nursing Outlook, 54,* 130–138.

Dracup, K., Cronenwett, L., Meleis, A., & Benner, P. (2005). Reflections on the doctorate of nursing practice. *Nursing Outlook, 53,* 177–182.

Finocchio, L. J., Dower, C. M., McMahon, T., Gragnola, C. M., & the Taskforce on Health Care Workforce Regulation. (1995). *Reforming health care workforce regulation: Policy considerations for the 21st century.* San Francisco, CA: Pew Health Professions Commission.

Fitzpatrick, J. J. (1989). The professional doctorate as an entry level into clinical practice. *Nurse Education Today, 25,* 222–229.

Fulton, J. S., & Lyon, B. L. (2005). The need for some sense making: Doctor of nursing practice. *Online Journal of Issues in Nursing, 10.* Retrieved January 10, 2008, from http://www.nursingworld.org/MainMenuCategories/ANAMarketplace/ANAPeriodicals/OJIN/TableofContents/Volume102005/Number3/tpc28_316027.aspx

Grace, H. K. (1989). Issues in doctoral education in nursing. *Journal of Professional Nursing, 5,* 266–270.

Hathaway, D., Jacob, S., Stegbauer, C., Thompson, C., & Graff, C. (2006). The practice doctorate: Perspectives of early adopters. *Journal of Nursing Education, 45,* 487–496.

Institute of Medicine. (2003). *Health professions education: A bridge to quality.* Washington, DC: National Academies Press.

Lenz, E. R. (2005). The practice doctorate in nursing: An idea whose time has come. *Online Journal of Nursing Issues, 10*(3). Retrieved June 18, 2008, from http://www.nursingworld.org/MainMenuCategories/ANAMarketplace/ANAPeriodicals/OJIN/TableofContents/Volume102005/Number3/tpc28_116025.aspx

Magyary, D., Whitney, J., & Brown, M. A. (2006). Advancing practice inquiry: Research foundations: Doctor of Nursing Practice. *Nursing Outlook, 53,* 139–142.

Oakland University School of Nursing. (2006). NRS 890 Syllabus. Rochester, MI.

O'Sullivan, A. L. (2005). The practice doctorate in nursing. *NONPF the Mentor, 16*(1), 1–2, 12. Retrieved June 18, 2008, from www.nonpf.org/newsletter.16.1.web2.pdf

O'Sullivan, A. L., Carter, M., Marion, L., Pohl, J. M., & Werner, K. E. (2005). Moving forward together: The practice doctorate in nursing. *Online Journal of Issues in Nursing,* Article 10913734, *10*(3). Retrieved January 18, 2008, from http://www.nursingworld.org/MainMenuCategories/ANAMarketplace/ANAPeriodicals/OJIN/TableofContents/Volume102005/Number3/tpc28_416028.aspx

Otterness, S. (2006). Implications of doctorate in nursing practice—Still many unresolved issues for nurse practitioners. *Nephrology Nursing Journal, 33,* 685–687.

Scholtfeldt, R. M. (1978). The professional doctorate: Rationale and characteristics. *Nursing Outlook, 26,* 302–311.

Yam, B. (2005). Professional doctorate and professional nursing practice. *Nurse Education Today, 25,* 564–572.

4

Doctor of Nursing Practice Clinical Experiences

CHERYL STEGBAUER

Highest-quality clinical instruction and evaluation of resulting outcomes are critical elements in Doctor of Nursing Practice (DNP) programs. This chapter focuses on the clinical education of DNP students and designing effective DNP programs with clinical experiences based on national association guidelines, chosen specialty areas, and institutional strengths. Discussion includes practical issues in clinical education, such as the development and evaluation of DNP clinical experiences in an environment with few DNPs in practice positions, as well as building on the culture and strengths of the university environment to develop clinical specialties in new DNP programs.

EARLY VISION FOR THE DNP: THE CLINICAL PERSPECTIVE

Twentieth-century visionaries responded to the need for doctoral level nursing practice in psychiatric nursing (Boston University, 1966; Farrell & Burgess, 1968; *New England Journal of Medicine,* 1963) and broader nursing practice (Christman, 1980; Fitzpatrick, 1989; Schlotfeldt, 1978). The 21st-century leadership of the American Association of Colleges of Nursing (AACN) and the National Organization of Nurse Practitioner Faculties (NONPF) was instrumental in moving the profession toward the reality of the DNP through ongoing national dialogue that led to the development of DNP standards and essential competencies. The DNP is a natural evolution of advanced nursing practice in response to unmet societal need (Hathaway, Jacob, Stegbauer, Thompson, & Graff, 2006). Just as early nurse practitioner programs transitioned from certificate programs to master's level education, the increased complexity and demands of high-level nursing care drove nurses to seek practice-focused doctoral education. Professional associations continue leadership with the development of specialty-specific guidelines supporting the DNP for advanced practice.

ASSOCIATION PERSPECTIVES ON DNP CLINICAL PRACTICE

The American Association of Colleges of Nursing

The AACN Position Statement on the Practice Doctorate in Nursing

The AACN Position Statement on the Practice Doctorate in Nursing is a defining document that provides insight and direction for the clinical practice of nursing at the doctoral level and for the development and conceptualization of clinical experiences in DNP programs:

> The term practice, specifically nursing practice . . . refers to any form of nursing intervention that influences health care outcomes for individuals or populations, including the direct care of individual patients, management of care for individuals and populations, administration of nursing and health care organizations, and the development and implementation of health policy. Preparation at the practice doctorate level includes advanced preparation in nursing, based on nursing science, and is at the highest level of nursing practice. What distinguishes this definition of practice from others is that it includes both direct care provided to patients by individual clinicians as well as direct care policies, programs and protocols that are organized, monitored, and continuously improved upon by expert clinicians. (AACN, 2004, p. 3)

This important statement recognizes the critical role and potential for doctorally prepared nurse clinicians and clinical experiences in direct care, policy leadership, and public health population-focused care. The subsequent Report of the AACN DNP Roadmap Task Force (AACN, 2006a) provides direction for faculty development and development and evaluation of DNP programs and clinical experiences.

AACN DNP Roadmap Task Force Report

All DNP graduates are expected to have attained master's level competencies for advanced nursing practice as well as DNP level competencies (AACN, 2006a). Thus, the variety of DNP faculty skills and credentials must meet advanced practice standards for faculty and clinical preceptors as well as provide for content areas such as health policy, epidemiology, statistics, and informatics. Accordingly, not all faculty in DNP programs are expected to hold the DNP degree. DNP faculty need the requisite skill and knowledge to teach their particular content area in the DNP program (AACN, 2006a).

The Roadmap report states that the scholarship of practice requires doctoral-level nursing faculty, and practice needs to be valued and recognized for promotion and tenure in universities (AACN, 2006a). Programs of faculty practice are essential to the mission of schools offering the DNP degree. A school of nursing that is part of a health science center may have cooperative agreements with faculty in medicine, pharmacy, or other health science disciplines to provide instruction in DNP programs and for interprofessional practice partnerships. Schools on liberal arts campuses may have access to resources in schools such as business and law. Faculty who are graduates of DNP programs will fill faculty positions as experts in their practice role and content, just as faculty in disciplines such as law, business, and medicine have educational preparation that focuses on the discipline rather than education (AACN, 2006a). AACN proposes that education should not be a major in a graduate nursing program; however, formal courses in pedagogy are desirable for nurse educators in addition to their specialty preparation (AACN, 2006a). Such courses are available through continuing education or other means. Table 4.1 provides the AACN Roadmap recommendations for institutions seeking to develop and support faculty for DNP programs.

The AACN DNP Roadmap Report (AACN, 2006a) identifies more than one educational pathway or entry point into the DNP curriculum. DNP programs are designed to accept students who have completed Bachelor of Science in Nursing (BSN) or Master of Science in Nursing (MSN) Clinical Nurse Leader (CNL®) professional entry programs

Table 4.1

AMERICAN ASSOCIATION OF COLLEGES OF NURSING (AACN): DNP ROADMAP TASK FORCE RECOMMENDATIONS FOR SUPPORT AND DEVELOPMENT OF DNP FACULTY

RECOMMENDATIONS FOR INSTITUTION

1. Require faculty teaching in the DNP program to maintain an active connection to practice in their areas of expertise.

2. Support individuals with a wide array of degrees and credentials as appropriate DNP faculty if they possess the needed knowledge and expertise.

3. Consider an exchange of faculty or faculty sharing between an established DNP program and a developing program as an approach to faculty development.

4. Engage faculty from other disciplines.

5. Recognize integrated scholarship as evidence for scholarship for the awarding of appointment, promotion, and/or tenure.

6. Support faculty with the DNP degree as eligible for appointment, promotion, and tenure if the institution tenures faculty with other professional doctorates.

7. Consider a range of appointment options to offer the greatest flexibility for employment and utilization of DNP faculty.

8. Develop education skills of DNP faculty.

RECOMMENDATION FOR AACN

1. Develop strategies for sharing "best practices" in the development of DNP faculty.

Note: From "DNP Roadmap Task Force Report," by AACN, October 20, 2006 pp. 15–16. Retrieved January 21, 2008, from htpp://www.aacn.nche.edu/DNP/pdf/DNProadmapreport.pdf.

in nursing and/or those who have completed MSN advanced practice nursing degree programs. It is important that as faculty admit to DNP programs and design clinical experiences, they consider the variability in existing master's level nursing programs. The DNP candidate's previous educational program must be evaluated when considering individual qualifications for DNP admission to determine whether the candidate's previous education included the learning experiences for master's level advanced practice competencies (AACN, 2006a). Admission portfolios that include documentation such as advanced practice specialty certifications are one method for evaluating competencies of individual post-master's applicants.

Candidates who enter a DNP program without advanced practice preparation will require a more comprehensive and longer program of study that incorporates master's level advanced practice competencies into DNP clinical preparation. The CNL-prepared DNP candidate brings competencies in evaluation and improvement of point-of-care outcomes as well as an understanding of health care systems' complexity and health policy in view of client issues surrounding accessibility, accountability, and affordability (AACN, 2007). The CNL competencies are consistent with some foundational competencies identified in *The Essentials of Doctoral Education for Advanced Practice Nursing* (AACN, 2006b). The DNP admission portfolio from the CNL MSN graduate might include examples of mastery of CNL competencies such as leadership in quality improvement at the microsystems level. The AACN DNP Roadmap Report identifies that AACN DNP Essentials 1–8 are the foundational DNP competencies for every DNP graduate. National specialty organizations further define the competencies, content, and practical experiences needed for each specialty (AACN, 2006a).

The Essentials of Doctoral Education for Advanced Nursing Practice

The AACN DNP Essentials are foundational outcome competencies that are inclusive of and expand upon master's level competencies (AACN, 2006b). The DNP Essentials report identifies that DNP education is by definition specialized, and that specialty content differs substantially depending on whether the specific specialty is as an advanced practice nurse focusing on individualized care or specializing in a practice role at a population, systems, or organizational level. Thus, competencies defined by the specific specialty organizations are a major component of the DNP curriculum. Specialty organizations develop the advanced practice competency expectations, content, and clinical experiences that build upon and complement the DNP Essentials 1 through 8:

1   Scientific underpinnings for practice
2   Organizational and systems leadership for quality improvement and systems thinking

3 Clinical scholarship and analytical methods for evidence-based practice
4 Information systems/technology and patient care technology for the improvement and transformation of health care
5 Health care policy for advocacy in health care
6 Interprofessional collaboration for improving patient and population health outcomes
7 Clinical prevention and population health for improving the nation's health
8 Advanced nursing practice

The DNP Essentials document notes that a final immersion practice experience is recommended to help students assimilate advanced practice knowledge at a high level of complexity to include a final DNP project. The final DNP project is a synthesis of the student's work in the DNP program and lays the foundation for future practice scholarship (AACN, 2006b). The final project is an outcome that reflects the practice focus of the DNP and is one method for summative student evaluation. The final product may take many forms while adhering to standards such as final review of the scholarly project by a DNP project committee advising and evaluating the student's project. Examples of projects include: report and documentation of an innovative practice change such as a quality improvement project; a manuscript submitted for publication reflecting the practice expertise and level of scholarship gained through the DNP program; or a practice portfolio documenting high-level advanced practice outcomes. Portfolios are one method to document case requirements, specific procedures, contact hours, and other required components of clinical experiences as a means of evaluating of clinical performance in DNP programs (NONPF, 2007).

Several resources for project development and templates are available to faculty and DNP students. The Virginia Henderson Library of Sigma Theta Tau International invites DNP graduates to submit DNP project abstracts for posting in the honor society's *Registry of Nursing Research* online database. Project submissions to the library can include scholarly activities such as clinical projects, health care policy changes, clinical outcomes/evaluation projects, translational research, and other projects to improved practice (Virginia Henderson International Nursing Library, 2007). Competency-based evaluation of learner performance and outcomes is a priority of health professions educators. A NONPF publication, *NP Competency Based Education Evaluation*

Using a Portfolio Approach, is the result of extensive development efforts by NONPF members and consultants (Beauchesne, 2007). The evaluation templates and portfolio rubrics include the doctoral-level NP competencies as well as the core NP competencies and provide a model with tools for competency-based evaluation of learner outcomes. The first edition of case studies published by Columbia University School of Nursing (2005) in conjunction with the Hope Heart Institute is an exemplar for evaluating student and program outcomes through the use of portfolios. The Columbia case studies publication was produced by the first faculty for the Doctor of Nursing Practice degree program. Students in the Columbia program are required to submit a portfolio as the capstone project. Case studies are a main component of the Columbia portfolio, demonstrating mastery of competencies. The portfolio also includes scholarship evidenced by peer-reviewed publication, presentations, quality assurance, and self-evaluation.

The DNP Essentials document identifies that faculty in DNP programs have the "academic freedom" to create innovative curricula to meet the competencies of the DNP Essentials (AACN, 2006b, p. 10). However, DNP programs preparing graduates in one of the four categories of advanced practice nursing (nurse practitioner, nurse anesthetist, nurse midwife, clinical nurse specialist) must prepare those students to meet eligibility requirements for national specialty advanced practice nursing (APRN) certification (AACN, 2006b). DNP program design and evaluation of DNP clinical experiences requires adherence to criteria determined by specialty organizations, including meeting quality standards and competencies for clinical preparation (Council on Accreditation of Nurse Anesthesia Educational Programs, 2006; NONPF, 2006b).

The DNP Essentials document provides further guidance for DNP program development and evaluation. DNP candidates who enter the DNP post-BSN, having met AACN BSN Essentials (AACN, 1998) would require a DNP program that is 36 months of full-time study; DNP programs are expected to provide a minimum of 1,000 clinical hours post-baccalaureate as part of a "supervised academic program" (AACN, 2006b, p. 19). However, the details of clinical requirements for DNP programs may vary according to the clinical specialty and requirements of certifying and accrediting bodies. Documents from nursing specialty organizations provide examples of guidelines for clinical education in DNP programs, including requirements for faculty preparation, supervision, and evaluation of clinical experiences.

National Organization of Nurse Practitioner Faculties

In 2000, the NONPF board identified a resurgence of the practice doctorate through discussions with early DNP adopter schools: the University of Tennessee Health Science Center; the University of Kentucky; and Columbia University (NONPF, 2005). NONPF leadership continued from that point to produce a series of presentations, formal discussions, entry-level practice doctorate competencies, recommendations for DNP student admission criteria and DNP faculty qualifications, and sample curriculum templates for doctoral NP education (NONPF, 2005; NONPF, 2006).

The Practice Doctorate Nurse Practitioner Entry-Level Competencies

The NONPF DNP competencies report was prepared by the National Panel for NP Practice Doctorate Competencies (2006). The panel membership reflected expertise in nursing education, NP advanced practice certification, program accreditation, and NP specialty organizations. Table 4.2 summarizes the DNP entry-level competencies for NPs.

The National Panel for NP Practice Doctorate Competencies (2006) further emphasized that DNP graduates prepared as nurse practitioners will possess the MSN level NP core competencies, including the skill to implement the full scope of practice as a licensed, independent practitioner, and that the doctoral level emphasis includes independent and interprofessional practice evaluating and providing evidence-based patient care across settings.

The National Task Force on Quality Nurse Practitioner Education (2002) was cofacilitated by NONPF and AACN with the goal to develop and refine criteria for evaluation of nurse practitioner programs. Task force members were leaders from 10 associations representing accrediting bodies and NP specialty certification organizations. The task force produced guidelines and standards for excellence and stability in nurse practitioner education. The criteria were then endorsed by 21 specialty organizations representing credentialing, regulation, and education of nurse practitioners (National Task Force on Quality Nurse Practitioner Education, 2002). A priority of the task force was to address and clarify criteria for clinical training of nurse practitioner students and the faculty resources needed for clinical oversight. The criteria are detailed and provide NP program evaluation criteria and evaluation templates

Table 4.2

NATIONAL PANEL FOR PRACTICE DOCTORATE COMPETENCIES: PRACTICE DOCTORATE NURSE PRACTITIONER ENTRY-LEVEL COMPETENCIES

I. Competency Area: Independent Practice

1. Practices independently by assessing, diagnosing, treating, and managing undifferentiated patients

2. Assumes full accountability for actions as a licensed independent practitioner

II. Competency Area: Scientific Foundation

1. Critically analyzes data for practice by integrating knowledge from arts and sciences within the context of nursing's philosophical framework and scientific foundation

2. Translates research and data to anticipate, predict, and explain variations in practice

III. Competency Area: Leadership

1. Assumes increasingly complex leadership roles

2. Provides leadership to foster interprofessional collaboration

3. Demonstrates a leadership style that uses critical and reflective thinking

IV. Competency Area: Quality

1. Uses best available evidence to enhance quality in clinical practice

2. Evaluates how organizational, structural, financial, marketing, and policy decisions impact cost, quality, and accessibility of health care

3. Demonstrates skills in peer review that promote a culture of excellence

V. Competency Area: Practice Inquiry

1. Applies clinical investigative skills for evaluation of health outcomes at the patient, family, population, clinical unit, systems, and/or community levels

2. Provides leadership in the translation of new knowledge into practice

3. Disseminates evidence from inquiry to diverse audiences using multiple methods

VI. Competency Area: Technology & Information Literacy

1. Demonstrates information literacy in complex decision making

2. Translates technical and scientific health information appropriate for user need

3. Participates in the development of clinical information systems

(Continued)

Table 4.2

NATIONAL PANEL FOR PRACTICE DOCTORATE COMPETENCIES: PRACTICE DOCTORATE NURSE PRACTITIONER ENTRY-LEVEL COMPETENCIES (*Continued*)

VII. Competency Area: Policy

　　1. Analyzes ethical, legal, and social factors in policy development

　　2. Influences health policy

VIII. Competency Area: Health Delivery System

　　1. Applies knowledge of organizational behavior and systems

　　2. Demonstrates skills in negotiating, consensus-building, and partnering

　　3. Manages risks to individuals, families, populations, and health care systems

　　4. Facilitates development of culturally relevant health care systems

IX. Competency Area: Ethics

　　1. Applies ethically sound solutions to complex issues

Note: From *Practice Doctorate Nurse Practitioner Entry-Level Competencies,* by National Panel for NP Practice Doctorate Competencies, 2006. In *Advanced Nursing Practice: Curriculum Guidelines and Program Standards,* by National Organization of Nurse Practitioner Faculties, in press. Washington, DC: Author. Retrieved February 1, 2008, from the NONPF Resource Center, http://www.nonpf.org/NONPF2005/ PracticeDoctorateResourceCenter/PDresource. Reprinted with permission from the National Organization of Nurse Practitioner Faculties (NONPF).

related to six areas: (a) organization and administration; (B) students; (c) curriculum; (d) resources, facilities and services; (e) faculty and faculty organization; and (f) evaluation. The evaluation criteria make explicit that nurse practitioner programs must have institutional support for faculty practice so that the lead NP faculty member and faculty members teaching clinical practica and clinical content are able to maintain certification in their advanced practice specialties and advanced practice licensure as required by state law.

The master's level advanced practice competencies are incorporated into DNP clinical preparation for the DNP (AACN, 2006a). Criteria for evaluation identify that to meet the NP program master's-level standards, a program must require a minimum of 500 supervised clinical hours; specialty tracks providing care to multiple age groups or that prepare NPs to function in multiple-care settings must require more than the 500 clinical hours. The number of faculty for direct and indirect supervision (coordinating clinical experience, interacting with preceptors, and evaluating students) is defined. The faculty:student ratio for direct on-site supervision is 1:2 if faculty are not seeing their own patients, and 1:1 if faculty are seeing their own patients; the faculty:student ratio for indirect supervision is 1:6 (National Task Force on Quality Nurse Practitioner Education, 2002). The NONPF Subcommittee of the Practice Doctorate Task Force (NONPF, 2008) identified that at some future point, all faculty teaching in DNP programs should be doctorally prepared. During the transition period from master's to doctoral programs, it is expected that master's-prepared faculty experienced in APRN education will be needed to teach in the master's-level portion of DNP programs. However, all courses, including clinical courses and clinical practica beyond the master's specialty level should be the responsibility of doctorally prepared faculty with specific qualifications reflecting the course responsibility. Faculty in clinical courses and practica at all levels must have current specialty certification (NONPF, 2006a).

American Association of Nurse Anesthetists (AANA): Report of the AANA Task Force on Doctoral Preparation of Nurse Anesthetists

The American Association of Nurse Anesthetists (2007) issued a position statement supporting doctoral education for entry into nurse anesthesia practice by 2025. Development of the AANA Position Statement and the Report of the AANA Task Force on Doctoral Preparation of Nurse Anesthetists (AANA, 2007) involved extensive input and study by association members. The decision to support doctoral education for entry represents the 75-year evolution of educational requirements for nurse anesthesia programs from hospital-based certificate programs, to university-based graduate programs in 1998 when the Council on Accreditation of Nurse Anesthesia Educational Programs (COA) required that all nurse anesthesia programs award a master's or higher-level degree (AANA, 2007). In 2004, the COA adopted standards for doctoral degree programs in addition to master's degree requirements (AANA, 2007).

Standards for master's level nurse anesthesia programs require extensive specialty content and clinical experience with an entry requirement of at least 1 year of experience as a registered nurse in an acute care setting (Council on Accreditation of Nurse Anesthesia Educational Programs, 2006). Master's programs must be a minimum of 24 months in length, with required courses and content in pharmacology of anesthetic agents, including chemistry and biochemistry (105 hours); anatomy, physiology, and pathophysiology (135 hours); professional aspects of nurse anesthesia practice (45 hours); basic and advanced principles of anesthesia practice including physics, equipment, technology, and pain management (105 hours); research (30 hours); and clinical correlation conferences (45 hours) (AANA, 2007; COA, 2006). Required clinical experiences in the nurse anesthesia curriculum include a minimum of 550 cases that represent a variety of required procedures, techniques, and specialty practice (AANA, 2007; COA, 2006). AANA developed competencies for the Certified Registered Nurse Anesthetist (CRNA) practitioner at the doctoral level that "complement the *Practice Doctorate Nurse Practitioner Entry-Level Competencies 2006*" (AANA, 2007, p. 196). Master's-level expectations and competencies of graduates include patient safety, perianesthetic management, critical thinking, communication, and the professional role (AANA, 2007). Competencies beyond the master's level provide a framework and basis for the practice doctorate curriculum for the anesthesia specialty. Table 4.3 reports the AANA practice doctorate CRNA competencies.

Association of Community Health Nursing Educators: Graduate Education for Advanced Practice Public Health Nursing: At the Crossroads

Members of the Association of Community Health Nursing Educators (ACHNE) voiced the need for guidance about graduate community/ public health nursing (PHN), particularly in view of the CNL as a master's-level generalist and the movement toward the DNP as the graduate degree for advanced practice nursing education (Association of Community Health in Nursing Educators, 2007). ACHNE leadership convened an association task force that explored and clarified the important issue of guidelines for graduate education for community and public health nursing. The 100-year history of PHN in the United States and the ongoing complexity of health care needs, including looming societal and global health threats, were additional drivers for the work of this ACHNE task force (ACHNE, 2007). The ACHNE task force recommendations were built on three assumptions:

1   The American Nurses' Association statement that public health nursing promotes and protects the health of populations using knowledge from nursing science, social science, and public health (American Nurses Association, 2007)

2   The Institute of Medicine (IOM) 13 content areas for public health science with endorsement of preparation in interdisciplinary practice (Institute of Medicine, 2003)

3   The AANC DNP Essentials of Doctoral Education for Advanced Practice Nursing (AACN, 2006b).

Table 4.3

AMERICAN ASSOCIATION OF NURSE ANESTHETISTS: SUMMARY OF COMPETENCIES FOR THE CRNA PRACTITIONER AT THE CLINICAL DOCTORAL LEVEL

I.   Competency Area: Biological Systems, Homeostasis, and Pathogenesis

  1.   Develops best-practice models for nurse anesthesia (NA) patient care management

  2.   Uses a systematic outcomes analysis approach in the translation of research evidence and data in the arts and sciences to demonstrate the expected effects on NA practice

II.   Competency Area: Professional Role

  1.   Demonstrates increased ability to undertake complex leadership roles in NA

  2.   Demonstrates leadership that facilitates intra- and interprofessional collaboration

  3.   Integrates critical and reflective thinking in leadership style

  4.   Demonstrates ability to utilize a variety of leadership principles in situation management

III.   Competency Area: Health Care Improvement

  1.   Uses evidence-based practice to inform clinical decision making in NA

  2.   Evaluates how complex organizations, public policy processes, and world markets impact the financing, delivery, and quality of anesthesia and health care

  3.   Develops, implements, assesses strategies to improve patient outcomes and quality care

IV.   Competency Area: Practice Inquiry

  1.   Assesses and evaluates health outcomes in a variety of populations, clinical settings, systems

  2.   Disseminates research evidence to diverse audiences through a variety of methods

(Continued)

Table 4.3

AMERICAN ASSOCIATION OF NURSE ANESTHETISTS: SUMMARY OF COMPETENCIES FOR THE CRNA PRACTITIONER AT THE CLINICAL DOCTORAL LEVEL (*Continued*)

V. Competency Area: Technology and Informatics

  1. Uses information systems/technology to support and improve patient care and systems

  2. Designs and uses information systems/technology to evaluate programs and care systems

  3. Critically evaluates clinical and research databases

VI. Competency Area: Public and Social Policy

  1. Advocates for health policy change based on excellence, ethics, cultural mores and values

  2. Influences statutory and regulatory aspects of health policy in relation to NA care

VII. Competency Area: Health Systems Management

  1. Demonstrates ability to analyze the structure, function, and outcomes of integrated delivery systems and complex organizations

  2. Negotiates, implements, and assesses business plans in a collaborative organization

  3. Develops and implements an integrated risk management plan based on information systems and technology to promote outcomes improvement for the patient, organization, and global populations

VIII. Competency Area: Ethics

  1. Applies ethically sound decision making for complex issues

  2. Informs the public of the role and practice of the doctoral-prepared CRNA and represents themselves in accordance with the *Code of Ethics for CRNAs*

  3. Fulfills the obligation as a doctoral-educated professional to uphold the *Code of Ethics for CRNAs*

Note: From *Report of the AANA Task Force on Doctoral Preparation of Nurse Anesthetists,* by American Association of Nurse Anesthetists, June 2007, Park Ridge, IL: Author.

Note: These competencies have been recommended by the AANA task force on doctoral preparation of nurse anesthetists. To the date of this printing, they have not been adopted by the Council on Accreditation for Nurse Anesthesia Educational Programs as a requirement for the accreditation of nurse anesthetist programs.

Table 4.4 compares the IOM content areas for public health science with the critical content areas for advanced practice public health nursing (ACHNE, 2007).

Direction for DNP programs with a specialty focus in public health nursing to provide care to populations is provided by three critical affirming statements from the ACHNE Task Force on Graduate Education. To advance public health as a specialty in nursing, ACHNE:

1 Supports the national movement toward the practice doctorate as a terminal degree for advanced nursing practice
2 Affirms the importance of and dedication to developing competencies for specialty-prepared advanced public health nurses using a nationally recognized process of competency development
3 Adopts the nomenclature of *public health nursing* to describe this field of practice (ACHNE, 2007, p 3).

The ACHNE proposes that doctoral nursing education with specialization in public health nursing is an evolutionary process that may include several pathways to the doctorate as the terminal degree. Collaborative models with schools of public health or other schools of nursing provide opportunities for program development and expansion. Further proposed is that educational standards and specialty competencies be developed based on the advanced-practice public health nursing content identified by the task force (ACHNE, 2007).

KEYS TO SUCCESS: VISION FOR THE FUTURE

The vision for practice-focused doctoral-level nursing education is at last a 21st-century reality. Not all graduate programs will immediately adopt the DNP, but DNP programs are the future of advanced-practice education in nursing in the 21st century. The NONPF board of directors envisioned that doctoral education will become the standard for entry into nurse practitioner practice as the DNP programs and practice evolves (NONPF, 2006b). Doctoral preparation should be a strong consideration of any future student considering advanced-practice specialization post-professional entry, or movement beyond previous master's preparation as practice-focused doctoral programs become available for specific specialties.

The practice options in existing DNP programs are exciting, with evolving specialties such as public health, family health, acute care and

Table 4.4

INSTITUTE OF MEDICINE 13 CONTENT AREAS OF PUBLIC HEALTH SCIENCE AND CRITICAL CONTENT AREAS FOR ADVANCED PRACTICE PUBLIC HEALTH NURSING

IOM PUBLIC HEALTH CONTENT	ADVANCED PUBLIC HEALTH NURSING CONTENT
1. Epidemiology	1. Epidemiology
2. Biostatistics	2. Biostatistics
3. Environmental health	3. Environmental health sciences
4. Social and behavioral sciences	4. Social and behavioral sciences
5. Informatics	5. Public health informatics
6. Genomics	6. Genomics
7. Communication	7. Health communication
8. Cultural competence	8. Cultural competence
9. Community-based participatory research	9. Community-based participatory research
10. Policy and law	10. Policy and law/health policy/ management
11. Global health	11. Global health
12. Public health ethics	12. Public health ethics
13. Health services administration	13. Leadership
	14. Population-centered nursing theory/practice
	15. Interdisciplinary practice
	16. Advanced nursing practice

Note: From *Graduate Education for Advanced Practice Public Health Nursing: At the Crossroads,* by ACHNE, October, 2007. Retrieved January 21, 2008, from http://www. achne.org/files/public/GraduateEducationDocument.pdf; *Who Will Keep the Public Healthy?* by IOM, 2003, Washington, DC: The National Academy Press.

critical care, psychiatric/FNP, forensics, nurse anesthesia, and health policy leadership. Delivery methods are state of the art with Web-based and Web-enhanced delivery of course content in many DNP programs in order to facilitate student access and to enhance doctoral-level education. Key nursing organizations will continue to review and refine criteria and guidelines for advanced practice and DNP programs for nurse practitioner preparation (National Task Force on Quality Nurse Practitioner Education, 2008) and other advanced-practice specialties. National specialty certification for advanced practice will reflect DNP preparation, both in changes to timing of when a student becomes eligible to take entry-level advanced practice examinations and in ongoing development of comprehensive board certification examinations for DNP graduates, such as the examination offered by the American Board of Comprehensive Care (2008).

DNP programs must acknowledge the lengthy and foundational preparation afforded by existing master's programs. Publications from national specialty associations as well as the American Association of Colleges of Nursing support acknowledgment and evaluation of previous academic progress in nursing as entré to the DNP. The competencies of MSN CNL graduates need to be acknowledged and documented as CNL programs become more common and the contributions of the CNL graduates are reported. Such acknowledgment may take the form of partnerships among universities, so that doctoral level programs may best partner with programs that cannot offer doctoral degrees but may prepare CNL generalists with advanced skills in safety and quality care or provide the courses that are now considered master's-level advanced-practice competencies that are foundational for higher-level DNP practice competencies.

Each school of nursing has unique strengths in view of the university mission, culture, history, and faculty qualifications. Building on those strengths is the key to planning a strong DNP program (Stegbauer, 2005). Evaluating the campus and regional culture and environment provides direction for new program development and helping existing MSN programs as they evolve to offer practice-focused doctoral education. Liberal arts and health science center campuses have different strengths for supporting schools of nursing with DNP programs, just as location in a particular state, region, or country may influence the mission to address the particular health needs of a population. Partnering with a school of public health to offer a DNP specialty track in public health or a DNP family nurse practitioner program with attention to the special needs and issues for delivery of primary care in rural or urban settings are examples of building on strengths and addressing the need for the highest level of nursing care. The development of DNP programs offers rich possibilities for interprofessional education and practice as well as best outcomes for patients. DNP capstone projects have the potential of setting standards for and providing evidence from the scholarly evaluation of care.

DNP graduates report the permanent and positive professional growth afforded by the practice-focused doctorate in their roles as nurse practitioners, nurse anesthetists, clinical nurse specialists, nurse educators, and nurse managers/executives in agencies that represent education, private practice, public health, acute care, primary care, and long-term care (Graff, Russell, & Stegbauer, 2007). Examining the impact of DNP care on patient outcomes and ultimately the nation's health is an essential goal for the profession.

REFERENCES

American Association of Colleges of Nursing. (1998). *The essentials of baccalaureate education for professional nursing practice.* Retrieved June 18, 2008, from htpp://www.aacn.nche.edu

American Association of Colleges of Nursing. (2004, October). *AACN position statement on the practice doctorate in nursing.* Retrieved January 21, 2008, from htpp://www.aacn.nche.edu/DNP/pdf/DNP.pdf

American Association of Colleges of Nursing. (2006a, October 20). *DNP roadmap task force report.* Retrieved January 21, 2008, from htpp://www.aacn.nche.edu/DNP/pdf/DNProadmapreport.pdf

American Association of Colleges of Nursing. (2006b, October 30). *The essentials of doctoral education for advanced practice nursing.* Retrieved January 21, 2008, from htpp://www.aacn.nche.edu/DNP/pdf/essentials.pdf

American Association of Colleges of Nursing. (2007). *White paper on the education and role of the Clinical Nurse Leader (CNL®).* Retrieved January 8, 2008, from http://www.aacn.nche.edu/Publications/WhitePapers/ClinicalNurseLeader07.pdf

American Association of Nurse Anesthetists. (2007, June). *Report of the AANA Task Force on Doctoral Preparation of Nurse Anesthetists.* Park Ridge, IL: Author.

American Board of Comprehensive Care. (2008). *The American Board of Comprehensive Care press release March 10, 2008.* Retrieved March 31, 2008, from http://www.abcc.dnpcert.org/pressrelease.shtml

American Nurses Association. (2007). *Public health nursing: Scope and standards of practice.* Silver Springs, MD: Nurses Books.Org.

Association of Community Health Nursing Educators. (2007, October). *Graduate education for advanced practice public health nursing: At the crossroads.* Retrieved January 21, 2008, from http://www.achne.org/files/public/GraduateEducationDocument.pdf

Beauchesne, M. A. (Ed.). (2007). *NP competency based education evaluations using a portfolio approach.* Washington, DC: National Organization of Nurse Practitioner Faculties.

Boston University School of Nursing Faculty Minutes. (1966, October 13). *Evolution of a doctoral program in nursing Boston University School of Nursing (BU SON).* Boston: Boston University Nursing Archives.

Christman, L. (1980). Leadership in practice. *Image: Journal of Nursing Scholarship, 12,* 31–33.

Columbia University School of Nursing. (2005). *Case studies for the doctor of nursing practice DrNP: Setting a new standard in health care.* New York: Columbia University School of Nursing in conjunction with the Hope Heart Institute, Seattle, WA.

Council on Accreditation of Nurse Anesthesia Educational Programs. (2006). *Standards for accreditation of nurse anesthesia educational programs.* Park Ridge, IL: Author.

Farrell, M., & Burgess, A. W. (1968). *The evolution of a doctoral program in nursing.* Unpublished monograph, Boston University Nursing Archives, Boston.

Fitzpatrick, J. J. (1989). The professional doctorate as an entry level into clinical practice. In *Perspectives in Nursing 1987–1989* (pp. 53–56). New York: National League for Nursing.

Graff, C. J., Russell, C. K., & Stegbauer, C. C. (2007). Formative and summative evaluation of a practice doctorate program. *Nurse Educator, 32*(4), 173–177.

Hathaway, D., Jacob, S., Stegbauer, C., Thompson, C., & Graff, C. (2006). The practice doctorate: Perspectives of early adopters. *Nursing Education, 45*(10), 487–496.

Institute of Medicine. (2003). *Who will keep the public healthy?* Washington, DC: The National Academy Press.

National Organization of Nurse Practitioner Faculties. (2004). *Recommendations for the nursing practice doctorate.* Retrieved February 1, 2008, from http://www.nonpf.org/cdrecommendations.htm

National Organization of Nurse Practitioner Faculties. (2005). *Timeline of NONPF practice doctorate activities.* Retrieved February 1, 2008, from http://www.nonpf.com/NONPF2005/PracticeDoctorateResourceCenter/timeline0605.htm

National Organization of Nurse Practitioner Faculties. (2006a). *Faculty qualifications, faculty development, and student admissions criteria relative to practice doctorate programs: Recommendations.* Retrieved January 21, 2008, from http://www.nonpf.com/NONPF2005/PracticeDoctorateResourceCenter/Faculty&StudentRecsFinal.pdf

National Organization of Nurse Practitioner Faculties. (2006b, October). *Statement on the practice doctorate in nursing: Response to recommendations on clinical hours and degree title.* Retrieved January 21, 2008, from http://nonpf.com/NONPF2005/PracticeDoctorateResourceCenter/BoardStatementOct2006.pdf

National Organization of Nurse Practitioner Faculties. (2008). National Task Force on Quality Nurse Practitioner Education. *Criteria for evaluation of nurse practitioner programs web version in review.* Retrieved March 31, 2008, from http://www.nonpf.com/NONPF2005/NTFCriteriaWebVersion0208.pdf

National Organization of Nurse Practitioner Faculties. (2007). *NONPF recommended criteria for NP scholarly projects in the practice doctorate program.* Retrieved July 15, 2008, from http://www.nonpf.org/NONPF2005/PracticeDoctorateResourceCenter/ScholarlyProjectCriteria.pdf

National Panel for NP Practice Doctorate Competencies. (2006). Practice Doctorate Nurse Practitioner Entry-Level Competencies. In National Organization of Nurse Practitioner Faculties (In Press), *Advanced nursing practice: Curriculum guidelines and program standards*. Washington, DC: Author. Retrieved February 1, 2008, from the NONPF Resource Center, http://www.nonpf.org/NONPF2005/PracticeDoctor ateResourceCenter/PDresource.htm

National Task Force on Quality Nurse Practitioner Education. (2002). *Criteria for evaluation of nurse practitioner programs*. Retrieved January 21, 2008, from http://www.nonpf.com/evalcriteria2002.pdf

National Task Force on Quality Nurse Practitioner Education. (2008). *Criteria for evaluation of nurse practitioner programs web version in review*. Retrieved March 31, 2008, from http://www.nonpf.com/NONPF2005/NTFCriteriaWebVersion0208.pdf

New England Journal of Medicine. (1963). Editorial: First doctor of nursing science. *The New England Journal of Medicine, 269*(2), 109–110.

Schlotfeldt, R. M. (1978). The professional doctorate: Rationale and characteristics. *Nursing Outlook, 26*(5), 302–311.

Stegbauer, C. C. (2005). *Keys to success: Preparing faculty*. Presentation to the American Association of Colleges of Nursing DNP Regional Conference, Houston, TX.

Virginia Henderson International Nursing Library. (2007). *How to use the website: Submit a doctorate of nursing practice project*. Retrieved February 8, 2008, from http://www.nursinglibrary.org/Portal/Main.aspx?PageID=4019#AddDNPProject

The Doctor of Nursing Practice Degree: Reaching The Next Level of Excellence

5

MOREEN DONAHUE

Nursing leaders looking for career growth opportunities that will enhance their ability to effect change at the highest levels of the health care profession will find the doctorate in nursing practice an invaluable resource.

As a nurse executive who has been engaged in health care leadership roles for most of my career, the advantages of holding a doctorate in nursing practice have been plentiful. As chief nurse executive at Danbury Hospital in Connecticut, I have been able to translate my advanced education into programs and policies that directly impact patient outcomes.

Most importantly, the degree has given me the professional tools and educational credentials to make high-level health care management and policy decisions as a credible and integral member of the organization's leadership team. It has broadened my career opportunities both clinically and academically, while enabling me to break new ground in nursing research and program development on a system-wide level.

THE VALUE OF ADVANCED GRADUATE EDUCATION

The need for nursing leaders who can effectively articulate key issues is crucial given the increasing complexity of health care today. Hospitals recognize the vital role of nursing in keeping patients safe and in delivering clinical excellence and patient satisfaction. Lengths of stay are shorter, and the acuity is higher—factors that make it critical for nurses to remain clinically current and use their judgment when evaluating patients. We need leaders to create an environment that supports nursing and nursing education.

I began to realize the value of earning a doctorate in nursing practice while serving as senior vice president for patient services at Greenwich Hospital in Connecticut. At the time, the hospital was working toward nursing magnet designation, and nurses were playing a greater role in top positions throughout the institution. But as the hospital's leading nursing executive, I felt I lacked the expertise to interpret research and determine if the results could benefit the hospital and inform evidence-based practice. I also realized that the doctorate degree was fast becoming the credential needed to hold a leadership position in the health care professions.

Faced with this knowledge, I was determined to go back to school to broaden my understanding of the underpinnings of nursing research. I started by taking a graduate level nursing research course at Case Western Reserve University (Case)—a move that confirmed my earlier sentiments that a doctorate in nursing practice was the best path to professional fulfillment and excellence. But like many nursing professionals, I could not leave my family or current nursing position in Connecticut to attend Case in Ohio full-time.

CREATING A NEW MODEL FOR GRADUATE EDUCATION

I knew I was not alone in trying to juggle the demands of a busy career with the need to hone my skills as a nursing professional with advanced experience and education. I also knew that as nurses we are part of a profession that looks at breaking down barriers, whether it is helping patients to access care or supporting nurses to advance their careers.

I approached the faculty at Case about the possibility of creating a new model for earning a doctor of nursing practice. What if the professors offered the classes on-site at Greenwich Hospital, enabling nurses to further their education without disrupting their family or professional lives? Case officials were extremely receptive about the novel approach, and together we designed a doctor of nursing practice program that now serves as a model at hospitals nationwide.

At Greenwich Hospital, the first cohort of students consisted of 18 nurses (advanced nurse practitioners, nurse managers, clinical nurse specialists, nurse executives). Case faculty held classes at the hospital for two weekends (all day Friday, Saturday, and Sunday). Students had the rest of the semester to complete their course work online, but all the didactic was done during that six-day period with faculty.

We tackled other potential stumbling blocks early in the process, as well. Some nurses worried about mastering statistics after being out of school for so long. To allay these concerns, we offered an introductory statistics course that laid the foundation for the graduate course, enabling nurses to pursue their studies with confidence. Returning to school with a group of peers provided a built-in support system for students to tap throughout the semester. The hospital also offered financial aid to defray tuition costs.

This DNP model was so successful that Case received a Health Resources and Services Administration (HRSA) grant to duplicate the program at hospitals and other sites in the United States, providing nurses the flexibility to earn the degree without leaving home or work. The model also highlights the value of forming partnerships that allow nurses in academic and acute-care settings to share resources and expertise. The university now offers graduate courses at off-site destinations—such as St. Kitts in the Caribbean—as a creative way for nurses to incorporate studies into their vacations. Danbury Hospital is using the model to bring master's and bachelor's level nursing programs on-site, as well.

Here are a few of the benefits for the nurse executive of holding a doctorate in nursing practice, based on my experiences as a 40-year veteran in the nursing profession.

EXPANDED CAREER OPPORTUNITIES

I became a special projects consultant with Bridgeport Hospital, where I continued my doctoral work in nurse empowerment and patient satisfaction. I was working with hospital leaders to establish a shared governance model and improve patient satisfaction.

I was not thinking about leaving my post at Bridgeport Hospital when a recruiter contacted me about joining the leadership team at Danbury Hospital as chief nurse executive. Having a doctorate in nursing practice differentiated me from other candidates and helped me to be selected for one of the most challenging and rewarding positions of my career.

On the academic front, I am educating future nurse leaders as a clinical faculty member for Case, Fairfield University, Sacred Heart University, and other institutions. Universities are hiring nurses with doctorates in nursing practice as faculty, some with tenure tracks. The current shortage of nursing faculty underscores the importance of developing a new cadre of doctorally prepared faculty.

TRANSLATING RESEARCH INTO PRACTICE

Understanding how to interpret research and translate evidence-based results into practice is an important skill, whether you are a nurse in private practice or work at a hospital or community health setting. At Danbury Hospital, my advanced education enabled me to evaluate nurse assessment tools and replace those with little validity with research-based instruments shown to make a real difference in patient outcomes.

As a member of the performance improvement committee for Danbury Health Systems, I guide staff by reviewing evidence-based practices and nursing-sensitive quality indicators and work with nurses and other caregivers to implement evidence-based practices to improve patient outcomes, including decreasing patient falls and preventing pressure ulcers. Implementing these measures not only enhances patient safety, but also contributes to the organization's financial stability. Beginning in October 2008, Medicare will no longer reimburse hospitals for care associated with preventable injuries.

BREAKING NEW GROUND WITH RESEARCH

Learning to conduct research that withstands peer review and helps nurse leaders improve patient care outcomes is another important benefit of the doctorate in nursing practice. Nurses gain practical knowledge on developing viable research proposals, from the importance of selecting theoretically based topics to understanding how to conduct a review of the literature. Soundly prepared research proposals have a better chance of funding and gaining approval from the institutional review board and other scientific review boards.

Again, these skills have proved invaluable at Danbury Hospital, where I have partnered with the chief medical officer to promote a culture of patient safety through a leadership-driven communication program. The interdisciplinary effort recognizes the contributions of all team members in relation to patient safety. I developed the research component of this program, entitled EMPOWER, which stands for Educating and Mentoring Paraprofessionals on Ways to Enhance Reporting of changes in patient status. The EMPOWER program is funded by the Donaghue Foundation.

As front-line hospital caregivers, paraprofessionals provide a significant portion of direct patient care, including vital signs, safety checks, and assistance with feeding, bathing, and toileting. Educating paraprofessionals to communicate changes in patient status may increase the number of rapid response team calls and result in earlier recognition of patient status deterioration. The EMPOWER proposal was selected after rigorous scientific review, because it could make a valuable contribution in the ability of staff to impact the delivery of care by recognizing changes in patient status early.

EDUCATION AND BUSINESS TRACKS OFFER PRACTICAL ALTERNATIVES

While a doctorate in nursing practice focuses on patient outcomes, the course work provides nurses with a broad view of the profession, including an in-depth look at nursing theory, health care policy issues, advanced nursing research, and other topics. Doctorate candidates can choose between two tracks: education or business management. This flexibility enables nurses to select a path that will help them improve patient outcomes based on their interests or employment. The clinical doctorate allows nurses to critically examine issues that are emerging in their institution or specialty.

For example, the health care policy course teaches nurses how to address national and state issues that could impact patient care at their institutions. I focused on proposed changes to visa requirements for nurses coming from Canada and Mexico to work in the United States. This was a major concern at Greenwich Hospital, where traveling nurses comprised a large percentage of the operating room staff. Recruiting and orienting that many nurses within the proposed visa time constraints would have been difficult. Thanks to the skills gained during this course, I was able to write a meaningful letter to congressional lawmakers, who eventually delayed implementation of the visa changes.

Students who choose the management track learn to develop business plans, a crucial tool for nurse leaders whether they are proposing new revenue-generating product lines, examining patient care delivery models, or assessing changing community health needs. This management track can be particularly helpful for nurse practitioners or other nursing professionals who do not have a business background. I pursued the education track, which included course work in curriculum development and a practicum with a mentor in teaching within the health care setting.

No matter what track you choose, all candidates must complete a thesis or a capstone project related to their clinical or private practice. I chose to do a thesis exploring the relationship between nurses' perceptions of empowerment and patient satisfaction using legitimate research instruments. Published in a recent issue of *Applied Nursing Research* (Donahue, Piazza, Griffin, Dykes, & Fitzpatrick, 2008) the study found a strong correlation between nurses' perceptions of empowerment and access to information, opportunity, support, and resources. The study showed a significant correlation between nurses' perception of empowerment and patient satisfaction.

MAKING A DIFFERENCE FOR PATIENTS AND NURSES

The theme of nurse empowerment resonates with many nurse leaders. I feel I have been empowered and energized since earning my doctorate in nursing practice. Whether it is examining health care policies or developing new patient care models, the degree provides nurse leaders with the resources and credibility to make significant contributions in the health care arena. It all goes back to the main reason so many of us became nurses: to make a difference in the lives of people who need our compassionate and skilled care.

REFERENCE

Donahue, M. O., Piazza, I. M., Griffin, M. Q., Dykes, P. C., & Fitzpatrick, J. J. (2008). The relationship between nurses' perceptions of empowerment and patient satisfaction. *Applied Nursing Research, 21*, 2–7.

6

The Clinical Nurse Leader (CNL)

MEREDITH WALLACE, SHEILA GROSSMAN, AND JEAN LANGE

The role of the clinical nurse leader (CNL®) was created in 2003 by nursing leadership at the American Association of Colleges of Nursing (AACN) to meet the needs of a failing health care system. (AACN, 2007). CNL programs are unique in that they are developed with identified, strong partnerships between both academia and health care providers, ensuring that the CNL educational programs meet the needs of the entire community of interest. CNL graduates are prepared to address the important health care problems of the future, including the needs of an aging population, chronic illness management, a growing uninsured population, and health promotion and disease prevention (Institute of Medicine [IOM], 2001).

CNLs may function as clinical change agents to improve patient outcomes by working with staff nurse cohorts. CNL graduates can address these needs as nonadministrative clinical leaders enhancing health care outcomes of patients in all health care settings, including acute care and community health settings. CNLs may also function as preceptors for CNL graduate students, as faculty at community colleges and in baccalaureate nursing programs, or as staff development educators who promote best nursing practices in health care agencies.

The purpose of this chapter is to provide a definition and overview of the role of a CNL. The chapter will begin with a discussion of changes within the current health care system that resulted in the need for the CNL role, including safety and economic issues as well as the need to provide care to rising numbers of chronically ill older adults with multiple comorbidities, uninsured Americans, and the impact of the nursing shortage on health care. Elements of the CNL educational program will be presented in relation to the specific health care needs the CNL role was created to address. A discussion of what the CNL role is and what it is not follows, including a comparison between CNLs, clinical nurse specialists, and nurse practitioners. The chapter concludes with a brief description of the day in the life of a CNL, and possibilities for the future.

A clinical nurse leader (CNL) is defined as a master's degree-prepared advanced generalist that puts evidence-based practice into action to ensure that patients benefit from the latest innovations in care delivery. AACN (2008) further defines the CNL role as:

- The CNL puts evidence-based practice into action to ensure that patients benefit from the latest innovations in care delivery.
- CNL are advanced generalists prepared at the master's level who serve as the "air traffic controller" on the nursing unit. The CNL serves as the central point of contact between the patient and other care providers, including physicians and nurse specialists. The focus of this role is clinical leadership at the point of care, not administration.

The CNL role was developed in 2003 by nursing leadership at the AACN to meet the needs of a failing health care system (AACN, 2007). The role is intended to provide a new model for care delivery that will positively impact the health care system by meeting the needs of patients, health care systems, and nurses. The American Organization of Nurse Executives (AONE) summarized the characteristics of CNLs as futurists, synthesizers, partners, conveners, provocateurs, designers, and brokers, who possess the values of creativity, excellence, integrity, leadership, and stewardship (Hasse-Herrick & Herrin, 2007). Bower (2006) described the CNL role as designed to address many issues and concerns related to patient care, including: (a) clinical knowledge, depth, and expertise; (b) critical thinking and problem solving; (c) the need for a strong nursing player on the interdisciplinary team; and (d) integrating evidence-based practice at the patient-provider interface.

The main role of the CNL is as a leader of the interdisciplinary care team and change agent within clinical practice settings. CNLs assume professional or salaried unit-based positions in which they identify unit-based problems; develop action plans to solve these problems; implement interventions in the form of patient care, education, and implementation of evidence-based practice; and evaluate the resolution of these problems. In so doing, the unit is compared against institutional and national standards to promote cost-effective care using primarily evidence-based practice. In this role, the CNL has the potential to make great improvements in patient care and the health care system. Essential aspects of the CNL role as defined by AACN are shown in Exhibit 6.1.

Exhibit 6.1

ESSENTIAL ASPECTS OF THE CNL ROLE AS DEFINED BY AACN

- Lateral integration of care for a specified group of patients
- Interpersonal communication
- Leadership in the care of the sick in and across all environments
- Design and provision of safe health promotion, disease prevention, and risk reduction services for diverse populations
- Provision of evidence-based practice
- Population-appropriate health care to individuals, clinical groups/units, and communities
- Comprehensive clinical decision making
- Design and implementation of plans of care
- Risk anticipation
- Participation in identification and collection of care outcomes
- Accountability for evaluation and improvement of point-of-care outcomes
- Mass customization of care
- Client and community advocacy
- Education and information management
- Delegation and oversight of care delivery and outcomes
- Team management and collaboration with health professional team members
- Development and leveraging of human, environmental, and material resources
- Management and use of client-care information technology

Note: From *White Paper on the Education and Role of the Clinical Nurse Leader (CNL)*, by AACN, 2007. Retrieved February 12, 2008, from http://www.aacn.nche. edu/Publications/WhitePapers/ClinicalNurseLeader07.pdf. Reprinted with permission.

AN OVERVIEW OF THE CURRENT HEALTH CARE SYSTEM AND IMPACT ON DEVELOPMENT OF THE CNL ROLE

A number of recent issues within the current health care system have played an important role in the need for and development of the CNL role. Specifically, issues concerning provision of patient safety in acute care facilities, the graying of the population as seen in the rising number of older adults who require complex nursing care, a capitated health care system that is facing limited reimbursement amidst rising health care costs, and increases in uninsured Americans place increasing demands on an already burdened health care system. Given the need for major reform in our health care system, it is hoped that the development of the CNL role will be a transforming force in addressing the following issues.

Patient Safety

Several regulatory organizations, such as the Joint Commission (2007) and the Institute for Healthcare Improvement (IHI) (2007) demand best practices in the hospital environment and are committed to holding hospitals responsible for patient safety. The Institute of Medicine (IOM) cites in their publication, "To Err Is Human: Building a Safer Health System" (1999) that 44,000 to 98,000 deaths per year in the hospital are due to medical errors and defines quality health care as "care that is safe, timely, effective, efficient, equitable, and patient centered" (IOM, 2001). The IOM recommended 10 new rules to redesign and improve care as a guide to improving care.

The Joint Commission's 2007 national patient safety goals delineate nursing's accountability to patients and families, including: encouraging patients' active involvement in their own care as a patient safety strategy, telling patients and their families how they can report concerns about safety and encouraging them to do so, and providing a written overview of all medications to patients upon discharge.

Research regarding improving patient safety (Aspden, Corrigan, Wolcott, and Erickson, 2004; Pronovost, et al., 2006, and Berwick, Godfrey, & Roessner, 2002) has increased attention to frequently identified problems regarding patient safety and has included recommendations for empowering nurses to practice more safely, and for monitoring various aspects of the health care system. Data-driven care will propel health care institutions toward a higher safety culture and, ultimately, improved quality of care. There is consensus that it is not just the people who interface with the patient, but the various parts of the system that provide the care (Porter-O'Grady & Malloch, 2007).

Nurses are in a unique position to provide quality care in acute care settings. In fact, the nurse, of all of the health care workers, has the highest number of contacts with patients and their families (Page, 2004). Because nurses are at the point of care they need to be involved in generating new ideas to promote patient safety, such as instituting a patient/family advisory board, developing safety initiatives on units that are specific to the patient population, marketing the unit and hospital's improvements in the local press as well as in the hospital, and offering safety best practices for the department or hospital. Impacting the safety culture of an organization is a challenging goal. By building a team with multidisciplinary staff and patient/family representation, and by linking these cohorts with the agency's board of trustees or a selected institution's governance body, it is believed that patient safety will be positively impacted. The CNL is uniquely qualified to identify what practices will generate the best patient care outcomes so that their unit or agency can become the benchmark for their system-wide facility or even other agencies.

Rising Older Adult Population

The United States is in the center of an unprecedented shift in the population. The Department of Health and Human Services, Administration on Aging (2008) reports that there will be 37.3 million older adults in the United States today, and that the number is expected to almost double by the year 2030. The result of this improvement in life span creates a vast increase in the number of older adults within the population. While older adults are healthier than they have been in the past, they tend to approach their last several decades of life with both acute and chronic medical illnesses in need of nursing care. Despite the increased needs of older patients, there is an international deficit in the number of registered nurses educated to provide this care. While the development and dissemination of geriatric knowledge and education has increased greatly over the past several decades, care of older adults in hospitalized environments is often less than ideal and in need of improvement.

Economics

The past century has witnessed extraordinary diagnostic and interventional improvements for care management in the health care system.

However, the sad reality is that much of the improved technology to detect and treat disease is not available to all patients because of the inability to pay for costly health care. In fact, the U.S. Center on Budget and Policy Priority (2006) reports that there were 46.6 million uninsured adults in 2005 (15.9% of the population) and 8.3 million children. This number represents an increase of 1.3 million uninsured adults in 2004 (15.6%). The percentage that is uninsured rose from 15.6% in 2004 to 15.9% in 2005. The number of uninsured increased from 45.3 million in 2004 to 46.6 million in 2005 (see Table 6.1). Moreover, the uninsured population, many of whom may be immigrants to the United States, often present with symptoms at a later date when the disease has progressed and is more difficult to treat, which presents extraordinary financial challenges to a capitated health care system.

Nursing Shortage

The Center for Health Workforce Studies reports that currently 30 states have shortages of qualified nurses, which results in an estimated 110,000 vacant nursing positions nationwide. The nursing shortage affects all areas of health care, including hospital units, community-based health care agencies, and long-term care facilities. As a result of this shortage, care provided at the bedside has been suffering. Nurses can only do so much in a given period of time. Aiken, Clarke, Sloan, Sochalski, & Silber (2002) report that for each additional patient per nurse, there is a 7% increase in the risk of dying within 30 days of hospital admission. A later study (Aiken, Clarke, Cheung, Sloane, & Silber, 2003) showed that a 10% increase in nursing educational level resulted in a 5% reduction in mortality of patients on the study unit, revealing that as the education of nurses increases, patient outcomes clearly improve. While the causes of the nursing shortage are multidimensional, the need to provide safe patient care is universal. CNLs, with a focus on unit-based patient care and safety, may achieve better outcomes with limited resources.

Need for Efficacious and Evidence-Based Health Care Delivery

The result of all this is the need to develop a health care system that provides efficient and effective care that meets patient needs. Efforts toward evidence-based practice (EBP), or "the integration of clinical expertise with the best available external clinical Internet-acquired

Table 6.1

HEALTH INSURANCE COVERAGE, 2001 TO 2005*

	UNINSURED		MEDICAID/ SCHIP	EMPLOYER-SPONSORED INSURANCE	INDIVIDUALLY-PURCHASED INSURANCE	MEDICARE	MILITARY HEALTH CARE
	Number (millions)	Percent	Percent	Percent	Percent	Percent	Percent
2005	46.6	15.9%	13.0%	59.5%	9.1%	13.7%	3.8%
2004	45.3	15.6%	13.0%	59.8%	9.3%	13.6%	3.7%
2003	45.0	15.6%	12.4%	60.4%	9.2%	13.7%	3.5%
2002	43.6	15.2%	11.6%	61.3%	9.3%	13.4%	3.5%
2001	41.2	14.6%	11.2%	62.6%	9.2%	13.5%	3.4%

*Based on Current Population Surveys. Percentages do not sum to 100% because some people have more than one type of coverage.
Note: From *The Number of Uninsured Americans Is Still at an All Time High,* by U.S. Center on Budget and Policy Priority, 2006. Retrieved February 12, 2008, from http://www.cbpp.org/8-29-06health.htm.

evidence from systematic research" (Sackett, Rosenberg, Gray, Haynes, & Richardson, 1996) is prevalent in nursing and other clinical arenas. In nursing, EBP uses a problem-solving framework to evaluate the published best evidence in the Cochrane Database of Systematic Reviews (http://www.cochrane.org/reviews) and evidence-based clinical practice guidelines of the National Guidelines Clearinghouse for evidence-based clinical protocols (http://www.guideline.gov/). This evidence is combined with the clinical expertise of someone like a CNL and applied to the patient's situation to develop the best practice for clinical plans of care (Melnyk & Fineout-Overholt, 2004). However, in any given nursing research class within which the importance of nursing research has been clearly ingrained, undergraduate, RN/BSN, and graduate students can all spontaneously identify examples of outdated clinical practice that is not reflective of currently available nursing research.

CNLs are not intended to replace clinical nurse specialists, nurse practitioners, or other advanced-practice nursing roles, but to complement these roles to promote improved patient care and health system outcomes. CNLs function as members of a team of nursing professionals designed to provide evidence-based care to patients in all care settings. Consequently, Harris, Tornabeni, and Walters (2006) suggest that strong communications between these members of the health care team may improve the intended outcomes greatly.

CNL EDUCATIONAL PREPARATION

Educational preparation for CNLs is at the master's level. Most educational programs require between 32 and 40 credits in a traditional master of science in nursing, with 400 to 500 clinical hours (300 of which should be an immersion experience). However, accelerated program options are available, and the CNL may be achieved within a post-master's certificate. Other educational considerations for the CNL education may be the direct entry into a Doctor of Nursing Practice program (DNP). The recommended CNL core includes elements of professional values, critical thinking, communication, nursing technology, and clinical management needed to prepare advanced generalists, such as health assessment, pharmacology, and advanced physiology and pathophysiology. While choices regarding the inclusion of this specific content vary by individual academic institution, the need to provide sufficient education to promote confidence and skill in clinical practice is essential. The core also may include a graduate-level research course, and health promotion content. AACN (2006) recommends that "all programs demonstrate achievement of the five IOM health professional core competencies: quality improvement, interdisciplinary team care, patient-centered care, evidence-based practice and utilization of informatics."

In order to provide efficient care to patients and to meet the complex needs of a changing health care system, CNLs are required to meet a number of competencies by the end of their educational programs, focused on the curricular elements of leadership and management of the care environment, along with clinical outcome evaluation. These competencies are outlined in Table 6.2.

CNLs require preparation in evidence-based knowledge and skills to maximize the development of using one's leadership potential in evolving and challenging health care systems. Thus, students must be educated to be creative, competent as decision makers, accountable, visionary, flexible, successful risk takers, managers of information and practice trends, change agents, conflict managers, and articulate communicators in the context of an interdisciplinary team. Leadership content must examine strategies that will empower nurses to become leaders in current and future health care settings, facilitating the formulation of a vision for creating nurse-driven protocols to lead health care providers in delivering quality, safe patient care. Moreover, educational programs may include opportunities to develop patient-focused goals using innovative and visionary methods to optimize outcomes for a specific patient population within health care organizations. Additionally, it is essential that CNLs be educated to develop strategies for leading nursing professionals in creating new ways of need prioritization and task delegation in order to enhance cost savings.

Management of the care environment includes the abilities to utilize database systems in order to enhance evidence-based practice and measure outcomes against internal and external systems. Thus, educational preparation in health care systems is essential. The need to understand nursing informatics gives CNLs the ability to utilize national databases to develop and compare unit- and system-based outcomes against national standards. Thus CNLs must be prepared in both health care systems management and informatics in order to effectively set and meet goals related to care management.

Table 6.2

CNL END-OF-PROGRAM COMPETENCIES

CURRICULUM ELEMENTS	END-OF-PROGRAM COMPETENCIES
Nursing leadership	1. Effects change through advocacy for the profession, interdisciplinary health care team, and the client. 2. Communicates effectively to achieve quality client outcomes and lateral integration of care for a cohort of clients. 3. Actively pursues new knowledge and skills, needs of clients and staff, and assists with evaluation of the new, evolving health care system.
Care environment management	1. Properly delegates and utilizes the nursing team resources (human and fiscal) and serves as leader and partner in the interdisciplinary health care team. 2. Identifies clinical and cost outcomes that improve safety, effectiveness, timeliness, efficiency, quality, and the degree to which they are client-centered. 3. Uses information systems and technology at the point of care to improve health care outcomes. 4. Participates in systems review to critically evaluate and anticipate risks to client safety to improve quality of client care delivery.
Clinical outcomes management	1. Assumes accountability for health care outcomes for a specific group of clients within a unit or setting, recognizing the influence of the meso- and macrosystems on the microsystems. 2. Assimilates and applies research-based information to design, implement, and evaluate client plans of care. 3. Synthesizes data, information, and knowledge to evaluate and achieve optimal client and care environment outcomes. 4. Uses appropriate teaching/learning principles and strategies as well as current information, materials, and technologies to facilitate the learning of clients, and groups of other health care professionals.

Adapted from *AACN CNL End-of-program competencies and required clinical experiences,* May 2006.

Clinical outcome management is an essential element of CNL education. To this end, CNLs assume the role of interdisciplinary team leader. Education focused on the identification of patient outcomes and the design of systems to effectively manage these outcomes is necessary. CNLs must learn to utilize leadership and management skills, manage patient outcomes, and demonstrate clinical competence through implementation of various aspects of the CNL role.

Finally, role acquisition and role transition content is essential to promote effective entry into practice, especially as early cohorts of CNLs establish the role in health care settings. Role content should include elements of the advanced generalist role of leader, change agent, clinician, teacher, consultant, researcher, advocate, collaborator, and clinical manager of microsystems. The change in role from baccalaureate to master's-prepared nurse should be analyzed by differentiating professional behaviors expected from new baccalaureate and associate degree graduates, experienced nurses, and CNLs. The CNL job description must be uniquely developed to include the essential aspects of the CNL role as defined by AACN. Special attention is needed to effectively develop advanced communication skills necessary for the smooth transition of the CNL role into clinical settings. Within educational programs students may conduct trend analysis on the history of master's-level nursing roles and their influence on individual care and health systems. Likewise it would be helpful for students to analyze the essential aspects of the CNL role as defined by AACN by developing case scenarios that reflect one or two of the CNL characteristics. For example, see Exhibit 6.2.

Following this, a transition focus is essential to facilitate the successful integration of CNLs into practice. The behaviors and skills required for these professional roles must be examined, with reflection on clinical experiences acquired throughout the educational program. Transitional issues, such as credentialing and liability, must be addressed. Role negotiation within the health care system is a focus of this educational preparation. It is essential that the preceptored clinical experience include an immersion experience of approximately 300 hours in length, usually given over the last 15 weeks of the program. Moreover, because of the systems focus of the CNL role, experts recommend orientation with various departments within the health care system, including pharmacy, risk management, patient safety, finance, and quality assurance (Rusch, 2006).

Exhibit 6.2

ROLE OF CNL: USING RISK ANTICIPATION AND DESIGN AND IMPLEMENTATION OF PATIENT CARE

The CNL on the Acute Orthopedic Surgical Unit at a large, urban teaching hospital designed a protocol for high-risk patients susceptible to Methicillin Resistant Staphylococcus Aureus (MRSA). The high-risk patients were diabetics, dialysis patients, immunocompromised patients with indwelling catheters or other invasive lines, patients from long-term care facilities, and patients with prior use of antibiotics (recent, within 3 months of hospitalization). The protocol included different intravenous and oral antibiotics, family and patient education on good hygiene, and two planned home-care visits by an RN post-discharge. The CNL had maintained records of patients most likely to contract MRSA and used this information along with evidence from the literature to develop this MRSA prevention protocol of care. All staff were educated, and outcomes in 6 months revealed 80% decrease in return hospitalizations for poorly healing wounds, 40% decrease in MRSA infections, and overall higher patient, family, and nurse satisfaction.

CNL programs are unique in that they are developed with identified, strong partnerships between both academia and health care providers. These partnerships have the capacity of ensuring that the developed CNL educational programs have clinical practice sites with which to do practice in the CNL role. In order to facilitate these clinical partnerships, the following questions may be helpful.

1   Who are the clinical partnerships in the community of interest?
2   Are they interested in employing CNLs? If so, on how many units?
3   Who will lead the programs from the clinical side? Who will precept students?
4   Will they provide students in the form of current baccalaureate RNs who are prepared for master's education? What is their timeline for completion and implementation of the CNL roles?
5   What resources can they provide in terms of teaching facilities, clinical faculty?
6   Will they provide support in terms of release time, paid clinical time, and scholarships?
7   What infrastructure is available to collect data to measure CNL outcomes both in the clinical and academic setting?

The end-of-program competencies of the CNL match well with AONEs Guiding Principles for Future Patient Care Delivery (AONE, 2004) in that AONE supports that the core of nursing is care and synthesized knowledge that is user- and access-based. Moreover, AONE's focus on nursing presence, relationships of care, and management of patient journeys illustrates the unique CNL role.

INTEGRATION OF THE CLINICAL NURSE LEADER ROLE INTO PRACTICE ENVIRONMENTS

Change is a constant in health care, and the integration of the CNL role requires much change on the practice side in terms of redesign of existing roles, functions, and processes (Bower, 2006). Bower further states that role clarity is essential in the integration of CNLs into the clinical environment. Thus, an understanding of what a CNL does and does not do is essential.

An important manner in which the CNL role may be clarified is through the use of a role acquisition course in the CNL curriculum. Through this route, CNLs may be educated, strengthened, and empowered to advocate for their role in health care settings. This will not only provide for the utmost work satisfaction early in the integration of the CNL role into clinical practice, but is essential to pave the way for successful CNL role integration in the future. But an important component of empowerment is accountability. Outlining what the CNL is accountable for is instrumental in effectively establishing this role in clinical practice. Moreover, documentation of the effectiveness in meeting the accountability initiatives will be the most effective measure of CNL success in clinical practice. The CNL is accountable for the health care outcomes of a cohort of patients, which impact the clinical and financial function of health care systems.

By utilizing the key curricular elements of nursing leadership, environmental management, and clinical outcomes management, effective health care outcomes will be accomplished. Successful education, delegation, and leadership are necessary strategies that will contribute to the value of the current health care system, which is struggling with issues of aging and uninsured populations in an environment of decreased resources.

CNL outcomes may be divided into various subcategories and may be measured as illustrated in Table 6.3. Harris, Tornabeni, and Walters

Table 6.3

MEASURABLE OUTCOMES OF CNLs	
Clinical	Numbers of infections Falls Medication errors Pressure sores
Financial	Staffing levels Direct care hours Length of stay Reimbursement Readmission
Functional	Activities of daily living
Satisfaction	Patient satisfaction ratings Nursing staff turnover (intent to leave)

(2006) report that preliminary evidence evaluating the CNL role reveals improvement in readmission rates, RN hours per day, and infection rates. The authors concluded that the assignment of CNLs to units within the health care system has been cost-effective.

SUMMARY AND CONCLUSION

After completion of the educational preparation and necessary clinical experiences as a CNL, students are required to take a certification examination offered by AACN in order to gain entry into clinical practice. The exam is offered four times a year by partnering schools of nursing. The 4-hour exam includes both multiple choice and simulated clinical questions. Results are provided within a few days after exam completion. Successful passage of the exam results in the issuing of a certificate by AACN. No state licensure in advanced practice nursing is available at this time. Recertification is required every 5 years.

The AACN Steering Committee CNL continues the work initiated by the Implementation Task Force (ITF) to promote improved integration of the CNL work on many levels as they work to improve patient outcomes. To this end, the steering committee is continuing to work with CNL partnerships to collect information on the number of CNL programs and students as well as CNL employment information and outcomes.

CNLs were developed to address many of the needs of a failing health care system. Graduates are prepared to address the important health care problems of the environments of care and will greatly impact many of the challenging health care problems of the nation, including the needs of an aging population, chronic illness management, health disparities associated with socioeconomic dislocation, and health promotion and disease prevention (Institute of Medicine, 2001). While the role is new, information is forthcoming to assist educational programs and clinical partners to develop CNL programs that will effectively produce graduates to fulfill their intended roles. While little data is available supporting the role of CNLs in clinical practice, available evidence is positive and, as more data is generated, the CNL role will become more clearly defined.

REFERENCES

Aiken, L., Clarke, S., Sloan, D., Sochalski, J., & Silber, J. (2002). Hospital nurse staffing and patient mortality, nursing burnout and job dissatisfaction. *Journal of the American Medical Association, 288,* 1987–1993.

Aiken, L. H., Clarke, S. P., Cheung, R. B., Sloane, D. M., & Silber, J. H. (2003). Educational levels of hospital nurses and surgical patient mortality. *Journal of the American Medical Association, 290,* 1617–1623.

American Association of Colleges of Nursing (AACN). (2007). *American Association of Colleges of Nursing white paper on the education and role of the Clinical Nurse Leader (CNL®).* Retrieved February 12, 2008, from http://www.aacn.nche.edu/Publications/WhitePapers/ClinicalNurseLeader07.pdf

American Association of Colleges of Nursing (AACN). (2008). *Clinical nurse leader (CNL®) talking points.* Retrieved July 22, 2008, from http://www.aacn.nche.edu/cnl/docs/CNLTalkingPoints.doc

American Organization of Nurse Executives. (2004). *AONE guiding principles.* Retrieved February 12, 2008, from http://www.aone.org/aone/resource/guidingprinciples.html

Aspden, P., Corrigan, J. M., Wolcott, J., & Erickson, S. M. (Eds.). (2004). *Patient safety: Achieving a new standard for care.* Washington, DC: National Academy of Sciences.

Berwick, D., Godfrey, A., & Roessner, J. (2002). *Curing healthcare: New strategies for healthcare improvement.* Hoboken, NJ: Jossey-Bass/Wiley Publishing.

Bower, K. A. (2006). *Designing a care delivery model . . . the what, the how, the CNL®.* Presentation given at AACN Regional Conferences on Clinical Nurse Leader, Denver, CO, June, 2006.

Department of Health and Human Services, Administration on Aging. (2008). *Statistics on the aging population.* Retrieved February 18, 2008, from http://www.aoa.gov/prof/statistics/statistics.asp

Haase-Herrick, K. S., & Herrin, D. M. (2007). The American Organization of Nurse Executives' guiding principles and American Association of Colleges of Nursing's Clinical Nurse Leader: A lesson in synergy. *Journal of Nursing Administration, 37*(2), 55–60.

Harris, J. L., Tornabeni, J., & Walters, S. E. (2006). The Clinical Nurse Leader: A valued member of the healthcare team. *Journal of Nursing Administration, 36*(10), 446–449.

Institute for Healthcare Improvement. (2007). *100K lives campaign.* Retrieved February 22, 2008, from http://www.ihi.org/IHI/Programs/Campaign

Institute of Medicine. (1999). *To err is human: Building a safer health system.* Washington, DC: Institute of Medicine.

Institute of Medicine. (2001). *Crossing the quality chasm.* Washington, DC: The National Academies Press. Retrieved February 22, 2008, from http://www.iom.edu/CMS

Joint Commission. (2007). *2007 national patient safety goals.* Retrieved February 22, 2008, from http://www.joint.commission.org

Melnyk, B., & Fineout-Overholt, E. (Eds.). (2004). *Evidence based practice in nursing & healthcare: A guide to best practice.* Philadelphia: Lippincott, Williams, & Wilkins.

Page, A. (Ed.). & Committee on the Work Environment for Nurses and Patient Safety. (2004). *Keeping patients safe: Transforming the work environment of nurses.* Washington, DC: Institute of Medicine.

Porter-O'Grady, T., & Malloch, K. (2007). *Managing for success in health care.* St. Louis, MO: Elsevier.

Pronovost, P., Holzmueller, C., Needham, D., Sexton, J., Miller, M., Berenholtz, S., et al. (2006). How will we know patients are safer? An organization-wide approach to measuring and improving safety. *Critical Care Medicine, 34*(7), 1988–1995.

Rusch, L. (2006). *The CNL® pilot at Hunterdon Medical Center.* Presentation given at AACN Regional Conferences on Clinical Nurse Leader, Denver, CO, June, 2006.

Sackett, D. L., Rosenberg, W. M. C., Gray, J. A. M., Haynes, R. B., & Richardson, W. S. (1996). Evidence based medicine: What it is and what it isn't: It's about integrating individual clinical expertise and the best external evidence. *BMJ, 312*(7023), 71–72.

U.S. Center on Budget and Policy Priority. (2006). *The number of uninsured Americans is still at an all time high.* Retrieved February 12, 2008, from http://www.cbpp.org/8-29-06health.htm

7

The Clinical Nurse Leader (CNL) Core

JOAN ROCHE, JEAN DEMARTINIS, AND ELIZABETH A. HENNEMAN

The clinical nurse leader (CNL®) was developed to meet the needs of a failing health care system (AACN, 2006). Graduates of CNL programs are prepared to work in all health care settings as clinical change agents to improve patient outcomes. With the assistance of AACN, CNL nursing programs throughout the country have developed CNL graduates that can address the needs of patients by leading interdisciplinary teams toward improved health care systems. This chapter will inform the development of future programs and provide an overview of the current evolution of advanced generalist curricula.

The creation of a new Clinical Nurse Leader CNL master's degree in nursing involved the simultaneous development of multiple new CNL curricula by many schools of nursing across the United States. The roadmap for these development activities was the CNL white paper (American Association of Colleges of Nursing [AACN], 2004b), and the CNL Curriculum Framework (AACN, 2004a). The CNL white paper, like the AACN (1996) Essentials of Master's Education for Advanced Practice Nursing provided a guide for the necessary elements of each curriculum. This paper was not prescriptive; it allowed each school to build its program in accordance with its own unique mission and vision.

This new master's degree, however, offered new challenges to the faculty developing the curricula. The AACN (2004a) CNL Curriculum

Framework recommended a shorter time frame than the traditional 3-year, 42- to 60-credit master's programs in nursing. The AACN recommended that new curriculum have a 12- to 15-month, 3-semester or 4-quarter time frame (AACN, 2004a, p. 1). The rationale for this time frame is the advanced generalist model, in which students do not need the course work or time to develop a specialist knowledge base. Although such a short time frame would allow schools of nursing to rapidly place new leaders in the delivery of health care, it clearly challenged schools to create curricula that met all the necessary competencies. This 3-semester time frame, with a maximum realistic course load of 12 semester credits, would translate to a maximum master's degree of 36 credits. Addressing the broad range of required competencies for the CNL (AACN, 2004a) in 12 to 15 months has initiated a variety of creative curriculum designs, as well as some potential pitfalls.

In addition to the short time frame, the nursing profession is facing severe faculty shortages (AACN, 2006) and competing demands on faculty time (Kauffman, 2007). Creating and teaching a new course is time- and resource-intensive. Thus, nursing faculty ask how they can integrate existing courses with new ones and still meet the AACN curriculum framework and time frame. Similar challenges and questions were faced by every CNL curriculum team in the United States. To capture a national picture of the various models and approaches to these challenges, the author reviewed the published graduate curricula of CNL programs associated with the AACN.

METHODOLOGY

Sample

To evaluate the state of the current graduate CNL curricula, Roche reviewed the CNL curricula of 59 schools of nursing listed in January 2008 on the AACN CNL Web site. Of these 59 schools, 13 were excluded for the following reasons: two did not have Web sites, five did not include a CNL curriculum plan or program of study on their Web site, and six presented only curricula as integrated course plans for non-nurses obtaining the entry-level master's degree. In these plans of study, the course work meeting basic nursing competencies could not be differentiated from those meeting master's competencies. After exclusions, the sample comprised 46 CNL programs of study.

Data Collection and Analysis

The required curricula were reviewed to identify the primary content area for each course, which was entered into an electronic spreadsheet. When a course title was not clear, the author clarified it by reviewing the course description, when available. Each content area was analyzed by frequency of occurrence and percentage of total sample. The results presented in this chapter represent analysis of the data published in January 2008. With any nursing program, curricula continually change based on many factors; however, the results in this chapter represent the curricula published on the AACN CNL Web site as of January, 2008 (see http://www.aacn.nche.edu/).

Organization of CNL Curricula

The curricular content reviewed in this chapter was organized into three basic categories: master's core, clinical core, and CNL specialty core. The master's core included course work required of all master's programs or concentrations within a school. The clinical core included content related to advanced management of illness. The CNL specialty core comprised all the remaining required course work that was beyond the master's and clinical cores.

The *master's core* was sometimes specifically identified by the school. To confer a master's degree, a college or university must meet the requirements of its parent institution, and the requirements of its individual accreditation body. These requirements may include the total number of credits, course work in specific areas, or specific thesis or project expectations necessary for a master's degree. As the faculty and their clinical partners developed the specific curriculum for each program, they were obligated to address all these requirements. The courses meeting these requirements were identified by some schools as the master's core and were required for all master's students in their school. This category generally included course work in research, theory, and statistics. The master's core of a few schools included course work in leadership, health systems, or policy. A course was included in this category if it was required for all nursing master's degrees (nurse practitioner [NP], master of science/master of public health [MS/MPH], clinical nurse specialist [CNS], nurse educator, nurse administrator, CNL, etc.) at the respective school.

The term *clinical core* was used by several schools to describe the content related to illness and disease management. The AACN CNL expectations for this content specifically state (AACN, 2004a, p. x): "All CNL graduates will have additional graduate level content that builds upon an undergraduate foundation in: Health Assessment, Pharmacology, and Pathophysiology."

For this analysis, the clinical core included course work in this content area on illness and disease management. The inclusion of this content in the CNL curriculum was discussed at length in early national meetings of CNL educators and service leaders. One question addressed at these meetings was whether all CNL students should take the same graduate courses in advanced health assessment, pharmacology, and pathophysiology as the NP and CNS students. The alternative model would be to develop specific CNL course work in this content area.

The *CNL specialty core* includes the required course work that is beyond the master's and clinical cores. These courses provide the knowledge, skills, and practice to prepare graduates for the CNL professional role. This organization of curricular content is sometimes used by schools that offer several master's degrees. All students are required to take the master's core, and certain groups are required to take the clinical core (typically NPs, CNSs, and CNLs). The remaining courses, for example, clinical practice time and specialty-related content, were specific for each concentration. Although CNLs do not have a "specialty" population, they must master a core set of competencies that represent the CNL specialty. These competencies, as specified in the AACN curriculum framework (AACN, 2004a), include outcomes management, care environment management, team coordination, health care finance, systems, and policy.

RESULTS

The courses were categorized into three core areas: master's core, clinical core, and CNL specialty core. Each course was characterized by its frequency (its appearance in a CNL program) and percentage of total sample (N = 46 CNL programs, see Table 7.1). Frequency was calculated if a course was required in the plan of study. Although most courses were three credits, the frequencies in Table 7.1 were not weighted by credit value. If the content was present in a program, its frequency was 1.

Clinical Core

Most programs (80%) required at least advanced health assessment, with 71.7% requiring advanced courses in all three areas of the clinical

Table 7.1

FREQUENCIES OF COURSES IN CNL PROGRAMS ($N = 46$)

COURSE	FREQUENCY (N)	PERCENT
1. Clinical Core		
Advanced health assessment[a]	37	80.4
Advanced pharmacology[a]	35	76.1
Advanced pathophysiology[a]	33	71.7
Advanced practice nursing	4	8.7
Combined health assessment, pharmacology, pathophysiology	5	10.9
Acute/chronic illness	5	10.9
2. Master's Core		
Research/evidence-based practice	46	100.0
Theory	33	71.7
Project	15	32.6
Epidemiology	14	30.4
Statistics	8	17.4
Thesis	6	13.0
Nursing science, scientific thought and inquiry	3	6.5
3. CNL® Specialty Core		
Clinical specialty courses		
Residency	46	100.0
Clinical course (not residency)	16	34.8
Didactic specialty courses from required framework		
Policy and health systems	34	73.9
Role	29	63.0
Leadership	24	52.2
Care (environment) management	16	34.8
Finance or financial management	16	34.8
Informatics	15	32.6

(*Continued*)

Table 7.1

FREQUENCIES OF COURSES IN CNL PROGRAMS (*N* = 46) (*Continued*)

COURSE	FREQUENCY (*N*)	PERCENT
Ethics	13	28.3
Health promotion	12	26.1
Health care quality/clinical outcomes management	10	21.7
Communication	5	10.9
Diversity/cultural competence	3	6.5
Population-based health care	3	6.5
Case management	2	4.3
Outcomes management/informatics	2	4.3
Change management	1	2.2
Required CNL® courses not directly required in the framework		
Program development	3	6.5
Teaching	3	6.5
Family and community	3	6.5
Program evaluation	2	4.3
Rural health care	2	4.3
Curriculum	1	2.2
Human resources and employee management	1	2.2
Natural alternative care	1	2.2

[a]In one CNL program, these courses were electives (published totals reflect only required courses).

core. This advanced content is required for master's education for all advanced practice nurses, including nurse practitioners, clinical nurse specialists, certified nurse-midwives, or nurse anesthetists. The Essentials of Master's Education (AACN, 1996) specifies that the content of the advanced practice nursing core curriculum "applies to *any nurse* prepared at the master's degree level to *provide direct client care*" (p. 12). The revised CNL curriculum framework recommended that "the CNL curriculum include three separate graduate level courses in each of the three content areas" (AACN, 2007, p. 30), both to develop CNL practice competencies and to facilitate articulation with Doctor of Nursing Practice (DNP) programs. These recommendations for three separate courses appear to be followed by the majority of CNL programs (71.7%). As a result, most schools require the same clinical core courses for CNLs as for advanced practice nurses (APRNs). CNLs are not considered advanced practice nurses, but they are nurses prepared at the master's level to provide direct client care.

Of the 13 programs (28%) that did not require all three graduate-level clinical core courses, 10 (21.7%) required a combination of advanced courses that addressed illness management, combined assessment, pathophysiology, pharmacology, and/or clinical management. Two programs did not require didactic course work in the advanced clinical area, and one program suggested these courses as electives beyond the CNL required courses. This important CNL content might actually be a thread in these programs or taught during the role or clinical course work. This approach would pose a difficulty for CNL graduates who decide to go on for a DNP. They would not be able to document adequate educational preparation in this area. One assumption of the CNL curriculum guide was "The CNL graduate is eligible to matriculate to a practice- or research-focused doctoral program" (AACN, 2004a, p. 1). Thus, lack of clearly documented course work in the advanced clinical core would require CNL graduates to take this course work as part of their DNP program of study. Given the shortage of nurses with advanced education, nursing faculty are responsible for ensuring that nurses who choose to advance their education will have a seamless path to their terminal degree. Nursing schools with CNL and DNP programs may be more focused on making the transition as simple as possible for nurses.

At the recent CNL national meeting (January 2008 in Tucson, Arizona) hosted by the AACN, nurse leaders discussed another potential issue related to this clinical core. The licensure of NPs and APRNs is well known to lack consistency across the United States (Christian, Dower, & O'Neil, 2007). Some states provide APRN licensure for nurses with a master's degree in nursing who can demonstrate success in the three advanced courses of the clinical core. This policy could be interpreted as valid for CNL graduates with the three advanced courses in the clinical core, allowing them to apply for a prescriptive license. This odd problem is not present in all states, but it clearly highlights the need for a consistent national standard for scope of practice at all levels. For the past 3 years, a national consensus process, involving over 25 national nursing organizations including NCSBN, has been working to develop a future

APRN Regulatory Model to address these inconsistencies. Within this new regulatory model the CNL does not meet the definitional criteria for APRN.

Master's Core

Research and Application of Evidence

In the sample of CNL curricula reviewed, some schools specifically identified the master's core for all their programs. Many schools did not reference this category. Whether articulated or not, at least one advanced course in nursing research was clearly a core element (see Table 7.1). All the schools reviewed had one or more courses in research- and/or evidence-based practice. This requirement is consistent with the AACN Essentials of Master's Education, which states that "separate or distinct course work in this area (*research*) is deemed essential" (AACN, 1996, p. 6). The CNL curriculum framework refers to evidence-based practice, rather than course work focused on research design. The approach or content of these courses in the CNL curricula varies considerably, reflecting a recent shift in the master's competency for nurses. The earlier focus was on master's-prepared nurses participating in the design and conduct of nursing research. The current focus for all master's nursing education is the translation role of "utilization of new knowledge to provide high quality health care, initiate, change, and improve nursing practice" (AACN, 1996, p. 6). This focus on the critique, evaluation, and application of evidence is consistent with the evidence-based practice competency described in the CNL curriculum framework (AACN, 2004a).

The titles of courses included in this research category and some course descriptions reflected mixed elements, from research design and conduct to evaluation and application of evidence (evidence-based practice). Some courses were generically titled "Research in Nursing," leaving to conjecture whether this title refers to design/conduct or evaluation/application of research. Other courses were more clearly titled and described, for example, "Research Design in Nursing" with a course description on the design and conduct of research. On the other hand, "Advance Evidence Application" was clearly described as a course on evaluating and applying evidence to practice. Some programs required two courses, one with a design/conduct focus and one with an evidence evaluation/application focus. Clearly, a program with only one required course focused on design/conduct of nursing research could thread evaluation and application throughout the program. On the other hand, evaluation and application could be overlooked. Accurate critique and evaluation of research evidence is an important skill for CNLs to apply appropriate evidence in practice. Clearly articulating this foundational skill in the curriculum, in both didactic courses and clinical practice experiences, would be essential for successful CNL practice.

Theory

A majority of schools (n = 33, 71.7%) had a required course in the theoretical foundations of nursing practice. This requirement is an interesting element in the curricula because it is not specifically required or recommended in the CNL curriculum framework (AACN, 2007). However, a course on theoretical foundations of nursing practice is included in the Essentials of Master's Education (AACN, 1996). Thus, the high percentage of schools including a course in theory likely addresses the master's essentials requirement. As providers and managers of care, CNLs must be competent to "use theory and research-based knowledge in the design, coordination, and evaluation of care" (AACN, 2007, p. 25).

Among the curricula reviewed, some course titles and descriptions reflected broad application of theoretical frameworks to nursing practice, including nursing and other theories. On the other hand, some schools required courses entitled "Nursing Theory," which were described as focusing only on theories developed by nurses. The CNL curriculum framework does not mention nursing theory but includes health care systems and organization theories (AACN, 2007, p. 32), theories on complexity, systems, and managing change. The theories required for CNL education could be taught in many courses, including systems, role, or leadership courses. A preferable theory course for a CNL program includes an interdisciplinary focus, integrating the rich theory base of nursing with that of other disciplines and focusing on the application of theory to improve practice.

Project and Thesis

Almost half (n = 21, 46.6%) of the programs designated specific credits to a project or thesis. More programs identified project credits (n = 15, 32.6%) than those identifying thesis credits (n = 5, 13%). This requirement may reflect the requirements of a parent university or school; if the university/school requires a thesis to confer a master's degree, a program is required to include a thesis. However, as in master's-level nursing programs nationally, this CNL analysis reflects the trend toward projects as the capstone requirement. This trend, in turn, reflects the change in focus of the master's-level research competency from conducting research (a thesis) to applying research (a project).

Slightly more than half (n = 25, 54.3%) of the programs did not designate credits to a capstone project or thesis. Although many programs referred to capstone projects as part of the residency or final clinical experience, any trend in the focus of these projects could not be analyzed due to insufficient detail in the published programs and course descriptions. The available descriptions referred to using evidence to design system changes for the population served in the final clinical or immersion experience. The CNL white paper does not recommend or require a specific project (AACN, 2004b), but these projects provide valuable evidence to document the accomplishment of "End of Program Competencies" (AACN, 2007).

One required element of the CNL curriculum is knowledge management, including epidemiology, biostatistics, and measurement of client outcomes. Most nurses with a baccalaureate degree have a required course in statistics. A recent statistics course (within the last 5 to 10 years) is frequently required for admission to a CNL or other master's-level nursing program. However, courses in epidemiology or outcomes management are not commonly required in undergraduate curricula. Epidemiology content is often included in community health or public health courses, but it is limited. Of the 46 programs reviewed, 14 (30.4%) required a graduate epidemiology/biostatistics course and 8 (14.4%) required a graduate statistics course. Measurement of client outcomes was frequently combined with quality measurement or outcomes management (see the following section on the CNL specialty core). The purpose of this content area is to ensure that CNLs have skills in interpreting and managing aggregate data. In this sample of CNL programs, less than half (44.8%) required course work in statistics or epidemiology/statistics. In programs without these required courses, it was not clear where students would gain statistical skills at the graduate level. Statistics is one area that is more difficult to incorporate as a thread within a program, as many nursing faculty members do not feel comfortable or qualified to teach statistical data management in didactic or clinical courses with other foci.

The last group of courses categorized in the master's core included three courses (6.5% of the programs) related to nursing science and inquiry. According to course descriptions, when available, these courses seemed to be master's-level foundation courses for progression to doctoral research programs. Although these courses may have valuable educational content, it is not clear that they are necessary for a CNL program.

The master's core was often shared with the other master's-level nursing programs sponsored by a given school. This overlap may explain the focus on research design or nursing theories, which are not elements of the CNL curriculum framework. The universal inclusion (in 100% of programs) of dedicated credits to research/evidence base for nursing demonstrates the strength of the commitment to a strong scientific basis for practice. This commitment reflects the current growth of new models to evaluate and apply evidence (Titler, 2004). Hopefully, with these new models, traditional research course work in some CNL programs can shift to the development of the skills necessary to apply evidence to practice. As the CNL movement progresses, it will be interesting to see if theory course work remains limited to nursing theories.

CNL Specialty Core

Course work not included in the clinical or master's core was categorized as CNL specialty core. In the 46 programs, the average credit hours devoted to the clinical core was 8, and the average credit hours devoted to the master's core was 9, totaling 17 credit hours for these two categories. This left 20 to 24 credit hours for the CNL specialty core, which showed the most diversity in its courses (see Table 7.1). This diversity is not surprising, as the course work in clinical and master's cores has been long part of master's programs in nursing. Since the CNL specialty core represents a new configuration of didactic content and clinical experiences, each school took a different approach. The most consistent categorization within the CNL specialty core was the clinical course work, including the immersion and clinical experiences integrated throughout the program.

CNL Clinical and Immersion Experiences

All 46 schools described similar immersion experiences in the last semester of the CNL program, reflecting the clear expectations provided in the CNL curriculum framework (AACN, 2007). The average credit allocation was 5.48 credit hours, which reasonably converts to the 300–400 hours required in the working paper (AACN, 2004b) and the most recent white paper (AACN, 2007). Overall, the immersion experience, residency, and/or capstone clinical experiences were the most consistently described elements across all programs. The immersion experience or clinical residency has often been a presentation topic at CNL partnership meetings and teleconferences. The clear description of the immersion experience in the CNL curriculum framework, and the opportunity for programs to share plans and experiences, resulted in structural consistency across all the programs.

On the other hand, more diversity was found in the clinical experiences prior to the immersion course. Of the course descriptions available online, a wide variety of approaches was represented. Some schools required specific clinical hours as part of didactic courses such as Advanced Health Assessment, Leadership, Care Management, or role courses. Other programs listed courses entitled Clinical Nurse Leader I, II, III, and IV, each with a clinical and a didactic component. Specific CNL competencies were taught and practiced in each course. A third group of programs listed one or more clinical courses entitled Clinical Practicum, Clinical Integration, or Clinical Role prior to the immersion experience. The curriculum framework expectation for clinical credits is a minimum of 400–500 contact hours, with 300–400 for the immersion (AACN, 2007). Therefore, the minimum required contact hours, prior to the immersion, is 100. Based upon this review, all schools met, and several exceeded the required minimum clinical contact hours.

The content area that varied most in this review of curricula was organization of the didactic course work in the specialty CNL core. Based on the curriculum framework (AACN, 2004a, 2007), three major groupings are required from 15 required components for the curriculum with 10 threads (see Table 7.2). The specified groupings are leadership (with 5 components), clinical outcomes management (with 4 components), and care environment management (with 6 components) and the 10 major threads. Three of the 15 components, illness disease management, knowledge management, and evidence-based practice, were required in the clinical and master's cores. The remaining 12 content areas and 10 threads were present in some form in the CNL specialty core. Faculty members and their clinical partners faced a creative challenge to determine which content areas would be taught in stand-alone courses and which would be integrated in CNL-specific didactic courses and clinical seminars. The short time frame required for this new master's program prevented schools from requiring dedicated courses for each content area with application in required clinical course work.

Table 7.2

AACN CNL CURRICULUM FRAMEWORK DECEMBER 2004. CNL CURRICULUM FRAMEWORK FOR CLIENT-CENTERED HEALTH CARE

NURSING LEADERSHIP

I. Horizontal leadership

II. Effective use of self

III. Advocacy

IV. Conceptual analysis of the CNL role

V. Lateral integration of care

CLINICAL OUTCOMES MANAGEMENT

I. Illness/disease management

- Care management
- Client outcomes
- Builds on and expands the baccalaureate foundation in:
  1. Pharmacology
  2. Physiology/pathophysiology
  3. Health assessment

II. Knowledge management

- Epidemiology
- Biostatistics
- Measurement of client outcomes

III. Health promotion and disease reduction/prevention management

- Risk assessment
- Health literacy
- Health education and counseling

IV. Evidence-based practice

- Clinical decision making
- Critical thinking
- Problem identification
- Outcome measurement

CARE ENVIRONMENT MANAGEMENT

I. Team coordination

- Delegation
- Supervision
- Interdisciplinary care
- Group process
- Handling difficult people
- Conflict resolution

II. Health care finance/economics

- Medicare and Medicaid/reimbursement
- Resource allocation
- Health care technologies
- Health care finance and socioeconomic principles

III. Health care systems and organizations

- Unit level health care delivery/microsystems of care
- Complexity theory
- Managing change theories

IV. Health care policy

V. Quality management/risk reduction/patient safety

VI. Informatics

(Continued)

Table 7.2

**AACN CNL CURRICULUM FRAMEWORK DECEMBER 2004.
CNL CURRICULUM FRAMEWORK FOR CLIENT-CENTERED
HEALTH CARE (*Continued*)**

Major threads integrated throughout curriculum

    I.   Critical thinking/clinical decision making
   II.   Communication
  III.   Ethics
  IV.   Human diversity/cultural competence
   V.   Global health care
  VI.   Professional development in the CNL role
 VII.   Accountability
VIII.   Assessment
  IX.   Nursing technology and resource management
   X.   Professional values, including social justice

Clinical Experiences in the CNL Education Program
The total number of clinical hours should be determined by the CNL program faculty. However, it is strongly recommended that:

- Each CNL student completes a total of 400–500 clinical contact hours as part of the formal education program.
- A minimum of 300–400 of these hours will be in an immersion experience in full-time practice in the CNL role with a designated clinical preceptor and a faculty partner over a 10–15 week period of time.
- The full-time immersion experience will include weekly opportunities with other CNL students, faculty, and mentors to dialogue on issues and assess experiences, particularly the implementation of the role.
- The immersion experience is in addition to the clinical experiences integrated throughout the education program.

In the programs reviewed, 23 different categories of didactic courses were part of the CNL specialty core. Many of these courses reflected the 15 components from the AACN curriculum framework. Only three categories (policy and health systems, role, and leadership) were represented in designated courses of at least half the programs (73.9%, 63.0%, and 52.2%, respectively). The remainder of this section on the CNL specialty core is organized according to the AACN framework: leadership, clinical outcomes management, care environment management, and major threads

Nursing Leadership

Nursing leadership is a major curricular category for the CNL, for which the elements of leadership are different from traditional views. One key difference is that CNLs are horizontal leaders who provide lateral integration of care. This model represents a less hierarchical structure than that for a leader with a formal position of power over a team, such as an administrator or manager. The CNL leads at the point of care, with a focus on clinical leadership, not formal management of equipment or personnel. Traditional formal leaders, managers, and CNLs have many overlapping skills. Team coordination skills, including delegation, supervision, interdisciplinary care, group process, handling difficult people, and conflict resolution (AACN, 2007) are similar for traditional leadership positions and for CNLs. Leadership courses designed to be taught across nursing programs and across disciplines traditionally include adequate content in team coordination. However, the concepts of horizontal leadership and lateral integration are clearly articulated only in leadership courses specifically designed for CNLs. When multiprogram or interdisciplinary leadership classes do not include horizontal leadership and lateral integration, students and faculty have to address these important CNL leadership elements elsewhere or risk missing these important CNL skills.

Care Environment Management

About one-third of the programs (n = 16, 34.8%) listed a required course in care (environment) management, one of the three major headings in the curriculum framework (see Table 7.2). All courses with this title were designed specifically for CNLs and were not taught to other nursing majors or disciplines. In some instances, these courses were combined with outcomes management, the third main heading from the CNL curriculum framework. In the curriculum framework, care environment management includes the six elements of (a) team coordination, (b) health care finance/economics, (c) systems and organization, (d) policy, (e) quality management/risk reduction/patient safety, and (f) informatics. Some care management courses were didactic/clinical courses with application of the six elements. Some were broadly described without mentioning the six elements. Several schools with a care management course that was focused on application required one or more courses with five of the six elements: health care finance/economics, systems and organization, policy, quality management/risk reduction/ patient safety, and informatics. No school required an individual course specifically in team coordination. Two schools (4.3%) required a course in case management, with some of the elements required in the care environment management area. No programs required courses in all six sub-areas. Each program with a care (environment) management course had a different focus, based on the required content in other courses.

Care Environment Management: Policy and Health Systems

A majority of programs (n = 29, 63%) required a course with content in Health Care Policy and Systems. Two of the six distinct areas within care environment management are Health Care Systems and Organizations and Health Care Policy. One program required a course in change management, a specific area of health care systems and organizations. The high frequency of these courses reflects a commitment to a strong foundation in systems and policy for CNL practice.

Many of these courses, according to a review of several graduate handbooks and course descriptions, appear to have been required across several graduate programs, including other nursing majors, public health, or combined MS/MPH programs, and MS/MBA (master's degree in business administration) programs. This approach allows CNL students to learn and interact with students from other nursing programs and disciplines. The course descriptions included content in systems and organizational theory as well as health care policy. The CNL system competency includes microsystems in health care, but in most cases the course descriptions did not clearly indicate if the required system courses addressed microsystem-level theory and application. The particular applications to microsystems could clearly be addressed in clinical seminars. The course descriptions offered little evidence of complexity theory, as recommended by the curriculum framework. This content area is a good example of the balance and tradeoffs accompanying each curriculum decision. Participating in courses with other disciplines and different nursing majors broadens the experience of CNL students. At the same time, some specific CNL content areas may be missing in a course broadly designed for several majors. This issue requires attention from the CNL faculty to ensure that the content is addressed elsewhere.

Care Environment Management: Finance or Financial Management

Only a third of the programs (n = 16, 34.8%) included a course on finance and financial management in health care. Of these, 13 programs included 3- to 4-credit courses dedicated to financial management, and three programs combined finance with health systems or policy. One course was on health services management and the rest were nursing courses that focused specifically on health care finance. Interestingly, the required finance courses were not from schools or departments of management or business. Health care finance/economics is a specific area of financial management including Medicare and Medicaid reimbursement, resource allocation, health care technologies, health care finance, and socioeconomic principles (see Table 7.2). In the programs without a course in finance (n = 30, 66.2%), the location of financial content was not always clear. Some programs described finance as part of a health systems course. A few programs included financial management in quality/outcome management courses, or with case management. A few programs did not have any clearly identifiable content in finance or financial management. The existence of a CNL position in a clinical setting often depends upon a strong analysis of the CNL outcomes, including cost-benefit. Because finance is not a strong element in baccalaureate programs, a consistent presence is important in graduate CNL programs.

Care Environment Management: Informatics

Informatics is one of the fastest growing areas in health care (Agency for Healthcare Research and Quality, 2006). Nurses are involved in evaluating and implementing informatics in health care systems. Informatics is one of the six sub-sections of the care environment management category of the CNL curricular framework (AACN, 2004a), but the latest white paper offers few details on the depth or content recommended in informatics (AACN, 2007). Of the 46 programs, 15 (32.6%) required a course in informatics. In the other 31 programs (67.4%), the titles and available course descriptions did not clearly demonstrate the location of informatics in the curriculum. In this specialty area, similar to finance, many faculty do not have extensive education or experience. Due to this shortage of informatics specialists in nursing faculty, it is understandable that all programs have not incorporated a full course in informatics. However, as informatics is one of the 16 identified CNL curriculum areas, as well as an important area for leaders in clinical microsystems, its lack of clear presence in a curriculum could be a problem.

Clinical Outcomes Management

Clinical outcomes management is the third major heading in the CNL curricular framework. Although many programs had specific courses designated in some part to clinical outcomes management, the presence of this heading area was less consistent than care environment management. Clinical outcomes management, as evident from the curricular framework (see Table 7.2), includes content categorized in the master's and clinical cores, that is, illness management (included in the clinical core), knowledge management, and evidence-based practice (part of the master's core). Twelve programs (26.1%) required courses in the fourth subheading of clinical outcomes management, health promotion. Some programs referred to health promotion, disease prevention, and management in course descriptions of the clinical core.

Ten programs (21.7%) listed specific courses with clinical outcomes management content and health care quality or quality improvement, 2 programs (4.3%) combined outcomes improvement and management with information technology, and 2 other programs (4.3%) combined outcomes management with care environment management. Thus, 14 programs (30.3%) required courses at least partially focused on the broad category of clinical outcomes management. In addition, 3 programs required courses in population-based health care, and the course description available included some aspects of clinical outcomes management. Clinical outcomes management was clearly incorporated in CNL programs in various ways, and some elements were present in all programs. The CNL framework was built with connections between care environment management and clinical outcomes management, and many programs may have crossover between environment management and outcomes management. It was not clear, however, from the programs reviewed whether mathematical and quality models (Dlugacz, 2006) were consistently present in all CNL curricula.

The AACN specified 10 major curricular threads: (a) critical thinking/clinical decision making, (b) communication, (c) ethics, (d) human diversity/cultural competence, (e) global health care, (f) professional development in the CNL role, (g) accountability, (h) assessment, (i) nursing technology and resource management, and (j) professional values, including social justice (AACN, 2007). When implementing these threads, educators always wonder who "owns" the basic principles for the thread. The presence of a distinct course for each thread in the curriculum ensures that its foundations are present and allows for solid application across other aspects of the curriculum. Of the 10 threads, 6 were clearly present in distinct courses. Critical thinking/clinical decision making and assessment were clearly articulated in the clinical core advanced health assessment. Four AACN-recommended threads were organized as distinct courses in the CNL specialty core in some CNL curricula, rather than threaded throughout the programs: (a) professional development of the CNL role ($n = 29, 63\%$), (b) ethics ($n = 13, 28.3\%$), (c) communication ($n = 5, 10.9\%$), and (d) human diversity/cultural competence ($n = 3, 6.5\%$). All four threads are important to the CNL, and their presence in the courses reflects the respective schools' commitment to each area. Ethics, communication, and human diversity/cultural competence are important elements required in all areas of nursing education.

On the other hand, the CNL curriculum builds on baccalaureate competencies. With a limited time frame for graduate elements, CNL programs have little room to repeat content expected from a baccalaureate graduate. The professional role thread, however, is different from the role of a baccalaureate RN, nurse practitioner, clinical nurse specialist, nurse educator, nurse administrator, or nurse researcher. Role was a focus that many programs included in required course work, rather than threading through other courses. The presence of threads in a curriculum often required analyzing the objectives of specific courses. Because course outlines were not available on published Web pages, this curriculum review did not include a detailed review of all of the threads. Therefore, the remaining threads (global health care, accountability, nursing technology and resource management, and professional values, including social justice) are not reviewed in this chapter.

CNL Role

The CNL is a new role, whose success will depend upon CNL students understanding the scope of this new role and differentiating it from existing roles (Spross et al., 2004). Thus, it is not surprising that the majority of schools created role courses ($n = 29, 63\%$), rather than incorporating it as a thread. Some schools had one role course, whereas others had a series of courses focusing on different aspects of role acquisition and role transition. Many programs articulated application of the CNL role as a key element in clinical course work. All program descriptions (100%) referred in some way to integrating the CNL role into some course work. Where course descriptions were available, role courses consistently included communication, ethics, and role transition from the baccalaureate role to the advanced generalist or leadership role.

Two programs presented an unexpected educational model related to the CNL role. Both schools had CNS and CNL programs, with identical course work required for both concentrations. The only difference in these CNS and CNL programs was two clinical courses (one initial clinical course and the clinical immersion course), which focused on developing and applying the appropriate role in each concentration. This model does not appear to address the differences between the two roles detailed by the AACN position (Spross et al., 2004).

One group of required courses present in 6.5% of the programs or less was not directly related to the CNL framework (see Table 7.1). Although these courses had titles that were interesting and valuable for master's-prepared nurses, they appear to have been included because they existed for other master's-level nursing programs at their respective schools. These courses included program development and program evaluation courses, which could have aspects of financial management, outcome management, and organizational systems. Similarly, teaching and curriculum courses could apply to health literacy and some areas of horizontal leadership. Rural health care would be applicable to nurses in a rural area to understand their population of interest, which differs greatly from an urban area. Although human resources and employee management or natural alternative care could be interesting electives, it was hard to understand why they were required elements of CNL curricula.

DISCUSSION

The specialty CNL core programs reviewed clearly represent a continuum. On one end, some programs were completely developed for the CNL. In these programs, all courses in the specialty core were new courses, with titles such as CNL practicum, CNL leadership, or CNL care and outcomes management. This sequence of course work culminated in an immersion clinical experience. On the other end of the continuum, some programs carefully chose existing courses from nursing and other disciplines (including public health and health services) to include the content areas required in the curriculum guide (AACN, 2004a, 2007). These programs also culminated in a specific CNL immersion experience. The programs in the first group focused on integrating the skills throughout the program, whereas those in the second group provided integration experiences only in the immersion. Most schools were in the middle of this continuum, combining new CNL courses with existing courses from other programs and disciplines in some areas; and integrating other curriculum elements in CNL role, CNL seminar, or CNL clinical courses across the program of study.

Challenges

As mentioned earlier, the shorter than traditional master's-level time frame for the CNL program was a challenge to all schools. Interestingly, most schools crafted their programs to meet the expectation of 36 to 40 credits. However, when sample programs were available, most were designed for 2 years full-time and 3 years part-time. These program durations did not address the AACN guideline to complete the graduate portion of programs in 12 to 15 months. The balance between creating new courses and creatively blending existing courses addresses the economies of scale needed to manage workload with the growing faculty shortage. Although the number of online programs was small ($n = 2$), such programs address the need in many areas without CNL programs. On the other hand, online education raises the challenge of articulation agreements with clinical settings and faculty supervision from a distance.

Pitfalls

Programs that required mainly existing course work, with a CNL immersion course to integrate all the CNL competencies, could fall into the trap of merely tweaking an existing program. This approach could entirely miss the demands and competencies of the new role. The CNL is not just a slightly different CNS (Spross et al., 2004). The same pitfall would occur when a program includes an existing nursing course in a CNL curricula, without any modification. Merely tweaking an old course in nursing research could miss the focus on evaluating and applying the evidence needed for CNLs. This reference to "old" courses was intentional. The new competency for all master's-prepared nurses is evaluating and applying research evidence rather than the "old" focus of design and conduct of research, which is now recognized as the role of the PhD nurse. Students taking a theory course focused only on nurses' theories may miss the necessary theoretical foundations for the CNL. Sharing courses with other disciplines and majors offers great benefits to CNL students in providing inter- and intradisciplinary experiences through the programs, but it is important to include the CNL focus as well as public health, administrative, business, or other foci. Facilitating the development of the CNL role could be very difficult for a faculty member from a discipline other than nursing or a nursing faculty person with little knowledge of the CNL scope and role.

"Custom" CNL programs with all new courses had some interesting pitfalls. Some programs included many 1- and 2-credit courses in each area. Developing and teaching such courses could become a nightmare in managing the teaching workload at a school with shrinking faculty resources. These "custom" programs infrequently included certain curricular elements, for example, informatics, skills in managing and interpreting health care quality data, financial management, health policy, and systems theory. If these elements are only integrated in role, clinical, or immersion courses, will these important competencies be overlooked?

Very few programs clearly published the relationships between their school and service partner(s) to reflect that the CNL model was developed by practice and education leaders. If the articulation between practice and education partners is not evident in the curriculum, this innovative foundation may not last. Online programs are particularly susceptible to this pitfall.

CONCLUSION

The CNL curricula reviewed here were developed by groups of faculty with a shared vision for a new nursing leadership role at the point of care. Both similarities and significant differences were evident across programs, suggesting that all programs will benefit from formal, systematic evaluation of CNL outcomes being conducted by the AACN. "One size fits all" has never applied to graduate educational programs in nursing or other disciplines, but CNL graduates need consistent and strong preparation in key areas, with preparation in other areas based on the needs of their specific populations, cultures, and systems. This consistent, strong, and need-based preparation is a key factor in determining the future impact of the CNL role nationwide. Maintaining the national dialogue among nursing leaders and ongoing communication among schools of nursing with CNL programs will hopefully refine CNL programs, allowing them to graduate clinical nurse leaders who achieve the goals established by the founders of this movement.

REFERENCES

American Association of Colleges of Nursing. (1996). *The essentials of master's education for advanced practice nursing*. Washington, DC: Author.

American Association of Colleges of Nursing (AACN). (2004a). *American Association of Colleges of Nursing preparing graduates for practice as a Clinical Nurse Leader draft curriculum framework*. Retrieved January, 2004, from http://www.aacn.nche.edu

American Association of Colleges of Nursing (AACN). (2004b). *American Association of Colleges of Nursing white paper on the role of the Clinical Nurse Leader*. Retrieved January, 2004, from http://www.aacn.nche.edu

American Association of Colleges of Nursing (AACN). (2006). *Faculty shortages in baccalaureate and graduate nursing programs: Scope of the problem and strategies for expanding the supply*. Retrieved February 23, 2008, from http://www.aacn.nche.edu/Publications/pdf/05FacShortage.pdf

American Association of Colleges of Nursing (AACN). (2007). *American Association of Colleges of Nursing white paper on the education and role of the Clinical Nurse Leader*[sm]. Retrieved February 18, 2008, from http://www.aacn.nche.edu/Publications/WhitePapers/ClinicalNurseLeader07.pdf

Agency for Healthcare Research and Quality. (2006). *Costs and benefits of health information technology: Evidence report/technology assessment*, AHRQ Publication No. 06-E006.

Christian, S., Dower, C., & O'Neil, E. (2007). *Overview of nurse practitioner scopes of practice in the United States—Discussion*. San Francisco: The Center for Health Professions.

Dlugacz, Y. D. (2006). *Measuring health care: Using quality data for operational, financial, and clinical improvement*. San Francisco: Jossey-Bass.

Kauffman, K. (2007). More findings from the NLN/Carnegie National Survey: How nurse educators spend their time. *Nursing Education Perspectives, 28*(5), 296–297.

Spross, J. A., Hamric, A. B., Hall, G., Minarik, P. A., Sparacino, P. S. A, & Stanley, J. M. (2004). *American Association of Colleges of Nursing working statement comparing the Clinical Nurse Leader and Clinical Nurse Specialist roles: Similarities, differences and complementarities*. Washington, DC: AACN.

Titler, M. (2004). Overview of the U.S. invitational conference "Advancing quality care through translation research." *Worldviews on Evidence-Based Nursing, 1,* S1–S5.

8

Clinical Nurse Leader (CNL) Clinical Experiences

JAMES L. HARRIS

The environments in which health care teams work are fragmented, complex, siloed, and require numerous handoffs, and patient stays have been compressed so services are provided in shorter periods of time (Begun, Hamilton, Tornabeni, & White, 2006). This creates opportunities for multiple errors to occur. One attempt to reduce care fragmentation and proactively manage patient care was the introduction of the Clinical Nurse Leader (CNL®), the first new role in nursing in over 35 years following the nurse practitioner. The CNL was developed by the American Association of Colleges of Nursing (AACN) in partnership with education and practice leaders (Tornabeni, 2006). The development of the role followed rigorous discussions with stakeholders and research on ways to enlist highly skilled nurses to engage in outcomes-based practice and improvement strategies. The CNL is a master's-prepared nurse who integrates evidence-based practice into action at the microsystems level to ensure patients benefit from the latest innovations in care delivery. CNLs function as generalists at the point of care and are prepared with advanced nursing knowledge and skills but do not meet the criteria for the advanced practice nursing (APRN) scope of practice. The role is not one of administration or management, but as a clinical leader who designs, implements, and evaluates patient care by coordinating, delegating, and supervising the care provided by the health care team. In order to impact care, the CNL has the knowledge and authority to delegate tasks to other personnel, as well as supervise and evaluate these personnel and the outcomes of care. Along with the authority, autonomy, and initiative to design and implement care, the CNL is accountable for improving individual care outcomes and care processes in a quality and fiscally effective manner (AACN, 2006).

EDUCATIONAL PREPARATION OF THE CLINICAL NURSE LEADER

Preparation of the CNL requires several components, including liberal education, professional values, core competencies, core knowledge, and role development. Liberal education is central to preparing the CNL and fundamental to success in the clinical immersion and future practice. This promotes critical thinking, clinical judgment, and ethical decision making. A diversity of thought and reason is evolutionary, as CNL students and those in practice master new skills and engage others to integrate various perspectives and divergent thought. A well-grounded liberal education helps ensure that practice is inclusive of broad-based knowledge. The liberal education is not a separate and distinct track of professional education, but a foundation for lifelong self and peer learning transformation. Program curricula vary; however, didactic and clinical immersion experiences must blend physical and social sciences, philosophy, the arts, and humanities. Some programs have particular focuses on economics, epidemiology, genetics, global perspectives, informatics, and communication. Regardless of the curriculum, the didactic and clinical immersion must be complementary, and experiences should build upon the skill sets and resources within health care systems.

As CNLs progress through programs of study and assume roles within a variety of systems, professional values and value-based behaviors are strengthened. Common values and behaviors germane to the CNL include: altruism, accountability, human dignity, integrity, and social justice. Socialization of others to incorporate values and behaviors into daily practice will be realized as more staff assume these roles and model behaviors for others, and the profession of nursing and other disciplines continuously endorse the role and realize the impacts generated by CNL actions (AACN, 2006).

The core competencies that all CNLs possess and use to direct practice are attained through graduate education. The competencies acquired range from a simple application to a more complex level of integration during clinical experiences. Critical thinking is an essential competency necessary for success as the CNL questions, analyzes, synthesizes, interprets, applies knowledge, and uses creativity to provide quality, client-focused, and accountable practice. Communication is another essential competency that requires continuous mastery of skills. Critical listening, quantitative skills, and verbal, nonverbal, and written communication form the foundation used by CNLs when assessing, intervening, evaluating, and teaching others. As therapeutic alliances are created, one is able to manage group processes to meet care objectives and complete responsibilities inherent in the role and functions. Assessment skills form the foundation of evidence-based practice. Risk assessments allow one to anticipate risks to patient safety and can be the basis for holistic assessments of individuals across the life span. Acquiring and using nursing technology and effectively managing resources underpins actions as the CNL designs, coordinates, and evaluates plans of care. An understanding of health promotion, risk reduction, and disease prevention is another competency that the CNL must possess as multifaceted resources are garnered in order for patients to maintain maximal functioning and well-being. The CNL also must possess knowledge of illness and disease management including pharmacology, pathophysiology, and symptom management across the life span, with emphasis on chronicity and sequelae of illness.

The constantly changing health care environment requires all providers to have knowledge and skills in informatics and care technologies. The CNL must possess advanced skills in order to discover, retrieve, and use information for evidence-based practice and effective health teaching. Effective CNLs must be able to identify potential and actual ethical issues that arise from practice and must be positioned to assist patients, families, and other health care providers with ethical decision making. The CNL must also be able to apply knowledge of human diversity and how variations affect health status. In a global environment, CNLs must understand the implication of sharing data across disciplines, cultures, and geographic boundaries. This is supported by understanding the economies of care, business principles, and how to affect change at the microsystem level. Another competency required of the CNL is using theory and research-based knowledge as care is designed, coordinated, managed, and evaluated. The final competency required for the CNL is understanding the role and responsibilities of a professional and leader in the health care delivery system. This requires development of personal goals, impact statements, and activities, and mentoring others in a variety of the professional nursing settings (AACN, 2006).

ASSUMPTIONS FOR CLINICAL NURSE LEADER PREPARATION AND PRACTICE

The successful CNL assimilates a vast array of knowledge and skills within the microsystem of care. Ten assumptions exist that guide CNLs to effect quality patient care outcomes (AACN, 2006). Each assumption is presented, with examples of how practicing CNLs or students during clinical immersions use them to successfully transition into the role and sustain innovative practice.

Assumption 1

Clinical nurse leaders practice at the microsystems level. A microsystem is the immediate setting in which patients, providers, support staff, information, and processes join in order to meet individual health care needs (Nelson et al., 2007). This requires the CNL to perform a needs assessment that includes patients and staff, and that consider the organizational politics and dynamics. Interdisciplinary team members and leaders within the organization must be included in the needs assessment in order to be prepared for any issues that could arise from individual desires and information these individuals have about the organization and future directions, especially those at the microsystem level. Based on the needs assessment, a plan of action can be developed that includes collaboration and buy-in from unit-based staff. Changes can follow and outcomes can be evaluated.

An example of the importance of conducting a needs assessment was quickly recognized by a CNL when reviewing productivity measures, slack time, and multiple missed opportunities in an outpatient clinic. Based on the needs assessment and data analysis, the CNL and clinic staff collaboratively developed a service contract for the clinic and communicated this throughout the health care system. The service contract outlined required tests and films to be ordered before a consult was entered into the automated system. Coordination and linkage of needs to skill sets and available time slots for service resulted, and the productivity metrics within the area rapidly increased. What were once multiple missed opportunities, whereby patient appointments were not open and workups were incomplete when a consult was ordered, shifted to additional appointment access, complete workups, and higher satisfaction scores by patients and staff. As a result of increased productivity, a cost-benefit analysis of recovering patients who had received mild sedation during procedures followed. Data revealed a number of patients served had multiple medical comorbidities and required additional assistance after procedures, with and without any sedation; thus, an additional position was funded by management for post-procedure intervention. This is one of many examples where the skills of a CNL are beneficial in collecting and using data to drive health care decisions and use of resources.

Assumption 2

Client care outcomes are the measure of quality practice. Improved clinical outcomes and financial stewardship within a unit or health care system are markers of success for the CNL. Central to outcomes and cost efficiency are reducing risks and creating a culture of patient safety. Clinical nurse leaders are educated to create and implement care plans that result in sustained outcomes and reduce risks. Data assimilation and communication of outcomes to staff in a meaningful and understandable way must follow in order for staff buy in and to celebrate successes. Numerous evidence-based data are available to staff, but it is the CNL who can review data and collaboratively develop policies and procedures that create avenues whereby positive change occurs and data trends are sustained. Observations and discussions with CNLs in practice evidence how risks to patients and costs can be reduced at the microsystems level.

A CNL assigned to a surgical unit was reviewing surgical infection rates with the interdisciplinary team and, upon further analysis and drilling down, discovered that each of the providers used a different pre- and post-operative protocol for managing total knee replacements. What followed was a review of outcomes literature that evidenced that specific protocols, if consistently followed by providers and treatment team members, could reduce risks and shorten hospital stays. The CNL, in collaboration with providers, nurses, and physical therapists, developed a standardized orthopedic protocol based upon evidence, and it was introduced for implementation by staff. Sustained results revealed a decrease in infection rates, shorter inpatient stays, and increased functional mobility of patients post-procedures. Thus, risks were reduced and cost efficiencies were realized. Another CNL assigned to an outpatient gastrointestinal (GI) area was reviewing the number of cancellations for procedures. Further analysis determined that patients who were insulin-dependent diabetics and scheduled for a procedure were canceling appointments or arrived for the procedure and required immediate intervention due to hypoglycemia. Using the expertise of the diabetes clinical nurse specialist, the physician, and the clinical dietician, a protocol and education plan for patients and staff related to pre-procedural measures to follow for insulin-dependent diabetics was developed and implemented. Cancellation and complication rates were reduced. A key component in this example is how CNLs recognize they are generalists as opposed to specialists and utilize the expertise of others to improve clinical and cost outcomes in individuals and groups within a unit or setting.

Assumption 3

Practice guidelines are based on evidence. Clinical Nurse Leaders are prepared with infinite skills in using evidence on which to base every aspect of practice. As clinical issues and demands occur at the unit level, skill in knowledge acquisition, working in groups, managing change, and disseminating new information to other health care professionals must underpin the actions of the CNL. The CNL must seek and apply evidence that challenges existing policies and procedures and ensure new evidence is embedded in practice. A CNL student assigned to an acute behavioral unit was asked by the staff to provide evidence that would support the development of a proposal to open a medical/psychiatric unit. Eager to succeed and build upon the confidence of the staff who requested the task, the student collected data that supported such a unit as well as opposing data. The student was mindful that the proposal would require input from both medical and psychiatry staffs, so meetings were convened inclusive of providers and support staff from each discipline when the data were being collected and subsequently presented during a case conference. Throughout the student's year-long clinical immersion, a proposal was crafted that was evidence-driven and inclusive of all parties. The result was an approved proposal to open a medical/psychiatric unit that eliminated the placement of patients diagnosed with medical and behavioral problems on a medical or surgical unit with one-to-one supervision for extended periods, and eliminated the problem of medical and psychiatric staff not developing a comprehensive plan of care to meet the biopsychosocial needs of patients. What began as a request to utilize evidence on which to base a decision resulted in mass customization of a cost-effective and patient-centered unit whereby two medical disciplines jointly managed a unit, interdisciplinary staff was engaged in the delivery of coordinated care, and patients' individual needs were addressed in a timely and effective way.

Assumption 4

Client-centered practice is intra- and interdisciplinary. For care to be client-centric the treatment team must mutually establish a course of action. Clinical Nurse Leaders must seek input from other team members when confronted with a patient issue and utilize available resources. This behavior must be consistently displayed and must set the stage for other staff to model. In a sense, accountability is being modeled, and other behaviors, such as participating in committees, getting staff involved in projects, and open dialogue with multiple disciplines, engender patient advocacy and coordination of care. A practice example is how a CNL and student assigned to an oncology unit recognized a potential issue and potentially averted an injury. An increasing number of patients were being ordered chemotherapy regimens on the identified unit; however, due to retirements and reassignments, only three of the registered nurses were certified to administer chemotherapy. This created numerous challenges to ensure that protocols were started and completed without interruption. As the coordinator of clinical care, the CNL and the student assigned for a preceptorship convened an interdisciplinary group of experts, and a unit-specific chemotherapy certification class was offered for additional registered nurses. As an outgrowth of the coordinated effort, the CNL student collaborated with the unit-based social worker, and an oncology support group began that included staff, patients, and families with great success.

Assumption 5

Information will maximize self-care and client decision making. In an age of technology, advances in genetics/genomics, and increased consumer demand for knowledge, CNLs are in pivotal positions to assist patients to construct genealogies and identify family patterns of health problems. Creating health literacy plans and information create opportunities for other care providers to guide patients, families, and communities to be health-literate. Information must be available, and units should have education champions that maintain current information, in turn fostering independence, health promotion, and disease prevention. In discussion with a newly assigned CNL, numerous information was available on a variety of health conditions; however, the information was outdated and written at an eleventh grade reading level. Working with the unit education champions, current information was developed at a level based upon the assessed educational level of patients and families, and daily educational sessions were incorporated into the unit activities.

Assumption 6

Nursing assessment is the basis for theory and knowledge development. Nursing assessments allow clinicians to capture data about available support systems, presenting health and social problems, and lifestyle dynamics that can be used as the basis of decision support. However, systems must be designed whereby the data can be stored and easily retrieved so that clinical improvements and interventions, continuous performance measures, and decision support technology are developed and updated. Examples of how CNLs have utilized nursing assessment data to advance nursing knowledge and develop clinical interventions include falls programs for stroke victims, prevention and management of hypertension in select populations, pain management in elders diagnosed with dementia, and diabetic follow-up and compliance. When one considers the impact that is driven by the assessment data, the CNL role can easily be justified.

Assumption 7

Good fiscal stewardship is a condition of quality care. With limited resources and in a competitive market, health care organizations must use personnel and material resources wisely and efficiently. The CNL must understand the context in which resources are managed, know the difference in fixed and incremental costs, identify the high-cost/ high-volume activities, and be able to compare costs nationally and across facilities. Beyond a basic understanding of business skills and organizational theory, the CNL must design strategies and programs that improve care while enhancing efficiency and the quality of care provided. Three examples illustrate how CNLs in health care systems were judicious in fiscal stewardship. A nurse manager requested the CNL to identify the number of one-to-one patient care hours used for elderly patients with a diagnosis of dementia. Finding that over 500 hours monthly were documented, the CNL developed a "sitter room" program whereby patients meeting established criteria were assigned to a dedicated room on the unit and staff were educated on the causes, risk factors, and precipitators associated with a patient being assigned a sitter. The CNL targeted six risk factors for intervention that included cognitive impairment, sleep deprivation, immobility, visual and/or hearing impairment, and dehydration. Sitter hours were markedly reduced, averaging approximately 35 hours per month as staff recognized precipitators and risk factors early and initiated interventions.

Another example of how a CNL leader identified a quality issue and considered how to avert potential patient complications and associated costs was related to spinal cord injury (SCI) admissions to the unit and nursing interventions. The unit was not a dedicated SCI unit, but a general unit providing medical, neurology, seizure lab, chronic ventilator, and cardiac telemetry services. Based on numerous patient complaints and inconsistency in the provision of care for SCI patients, a comprehensive SCI competency module for staff was developed and implemented. Care outcomes were improved, complications were reduced, and patients were more satisfied following the module implementation. In another example, a CNL was asked to lead a work group that reviewed what tasks registered nurses (RNs) had assumed could be completed by other staff. The CNL utilized principles from organizational development and systems redesign to guide the group to identify the tasks and frame strategies to align work to assigned staff within the organization. Multiple changes followed whereby functions were assigned to other staff and RNs had additional time to provide direct care.

Assumption 8

Social justice is an essential nursing value. The value of social justice is particularly significant for the CNL as it is directly related to disparities in health and health care. As CNLs work with vulnerable populations and communities at large, many of the basic tenets of community nursing must be used as assessments and implementation strategies are employed to address disparities. A CNL working with individuals diagnosed with mental disabilities and their families met with the treating team in a community setting and redesigned processes whereby access to care was readily available by carving out slots for acute visits secondary to behavioral exacerbations. Historically, these individuals were assigned a number in the queue for the next available appointment, often resulting in emergency room visits after hours and admissions to acute behavioral units, when only an outpatient visit was necessary. Another CNL working in a long-term care setting developed several interventions that enhanced socialization for bedfast residents by working with social services, rehabilitation medicine, and physical therapy to purchase assistive devices and equipment so that these residents could be out of bed interacting with others, such as community dining and scheduled daily activities. The CNL commented to staff that one must consider what it means to be bedfast with limited interaction with others and the numerous social and physical complications that can occur.

Assumption 9

Communication technology will facilitate the continuity and comprehensiveness of care. Use of distant and varied technology has greatly reduced the number of visits to health care providers. Technology that is designed to monitor patients' progress in the home and assisted living areas has proven advantageous, especially for CNLs in rural areas. For example, a CNL in a rural area has utilized technology for daily monitoring of blood pressure and blood sugar levels for patients in the acute and chronic phases of their conditions. Patients do not travel to a health care setting unless acute distress is evident. Electronic monitoring of compliance and conditions promotes care continuity and a comprehensive approach to care where the patient and family members are engaged in self-care practices. Another example of the benefits of technology is how a CNL utilized available resources to electronically capture interventions and subsequent successes. Disease- and diagnostic-related grouping outcomes data were extracted and trended that evidenced multiple interventions since the CNL started in the role. This information proved useful in justifying the role and provided the basis for employing an additional CNL on the unit. And a final example is how the CNL assigned to a stroke rehabilitation unit worked closely with a physical therapist to use camera telephones to validate transfer from a bed to a wheelchair for post-stroke patients who had returned to the home environment. If deficits were evident, home visits followed for additional education. As technology continues to expand, all health care staff must master and use options available that will limit return visits to an overburdened health care arena.

Assumption 10

The CNL must assume guardianship for the nursing profession. Establishing professional goals and strategies to assist all nurses to protect and promote the health of citizens and communities is a key function of the CNL. As the CNL role becomes more commonplace in health care settings, behaviors will be modeled that other nursing staff replicate, and leadership positions in professional organizations and healthier communities of practice can be created and sustained. Comments from CNLs after the role was fully implemented in settings have focused on their participation with faculty members in writing for publication, grant writing, assuming leadership roles on local and regional committees, and presentations at national conferences.

SUSTAINING THE CLINICAL NURSE LEADER ROLE

The dynamic nature of the health care industry, changes generated by external regulatory agencies, stakeholder demands, and health care innovations require that mechanisms be in place to modify care processes and skill sets in response to emerging needs. The success of the CNL role to date is credited to health care systems that recognized the need to redesign the care delivery model, hence reducing fragmentation of care and introducing tactics to increase continuity of care. Pivotal to the success has been the chief nurse executive in the organization, who became the champion and collaboratively designed markers of success that included input from academic partners and all stakeholders. The islands of improvement created by introduction of the role created a synergy of innovation and diffusion. The needs of health care systems and patients, coupled with the talents of faculty and staff, have created a shared vision of continuous improvement. The staccato pace experienced in units prior to the introduction of a CNL is now a melody of ordered and sequenced care delivery that benefits both the patient and staff delivering care. Sustaining the role will require ongoing commitment and championing by nurse leaders and academic partners. As CNLs are employed and transition comfortably into the role, portfolios of their successes must be built and communicated widely. The quantitative data will support additional positions to be funded. The rich stories of CNL outcomes communicated by staff and patients will be equally important when justifying additional positions.

SUMMARY AND FUTURE DIRECTIONS

Health care is at a critical crossroad. Multiple drivers and forces have created a complex situation whereby nursing must be poised to act and not react. The complexity of health care creates opportunities for nursing to continuously impact change and redesign systems of care delivery. The CNL role is a promising role, and ongoing efforts by clinical and academic partners can morph into standardized practices in which the health of citizens and communities can be protected and promoted. The health care arena is changing daily, and the technological advances will force systems to continuously address the best way to meet patient demands and needs. This chapter has provided an overview of CNL educational preparation, assumptions for practice and education, and examples that highlight the positive outcomes as the role has been adopted in health care settings across the country. The journey for CNLs has begun and is a promising dimension of health care quality and performance as care is coordinated and less fragmented.

REFERENCES

American Association of Colleges of Nursing (AACN). (2006). *American Association of Colleges of Nursing white paper on the education and role of the Clinical Nurse Leader (CNL®)*. Retrieved February 12, 2008, from http://www.aacn.nche.edu/Publications/WhitePapers/ClinicalNurseLeader07.pdf

Begun, J. W., Hamilton, J. A., Tornabeni, J., & White, K. R. (2006). Opportunities for improving patient care through lateral integration: The clinical nurse leader. *Journal of Healthcare Management, 51*(1), 19–25.

Nelson, E. C., Batalden, P. B., Huber, T. P., Johnson, J. K., Godfrey, M. M., Headrick, L. A., & Wasson, J. H. (2007). Success characteristics of high-performing microsystems. In E. C. Nelson, P. B. Batalden, & M. M. Godfrey (Eds.), *Quality by design: A clinical microsystems approach* (pp. 3–33). San Francisco: Jossey-Bass.

Tornabeni, J. (2006). The evolution of a revolution in nursing. *Journal of Nursing Administration, 36*(1), 3–6.

9

Building and Adapting Current Graduate Programs Into Clinical Nurse Leader (CNL) Programs

MARIANNE BAERNHOLDT, KATHRYN REID, AND PAMELA D. DENNISON

Traditionally graduate education in nursing has focused on the clinical role or the administrator role; however, because of the increasing nursing shortage and increased complexities of the health care system, new graduate roles are needed (Institute of Medicine [IOM], 2003). Nursing educational programs need to attract individuals into the profession who will provide clinical leadership in the health care setting (Radmzyminski, 2005). This does not mean there is a decreased need or support for nurses with advanced clinical skills but that there is also an emerging need for nurses to manage care on a microsystem level.

Beginning in 2000 the American Association of Colleges of Nursing (AACN) decided that a thorough report on nursing education, regulation, and practice issues was needed. The AACN board created two task forces: *Task Force on the Hallmarks of Professional Practice Environment* and *Task Force on Education and Regulation for Professional Nursing Practice*. Both of these task forces found that there was a need to change practice environments and nursing education (Tornabeni, 2006). Input and consultation was sought from AACN members, nursing practice leaders, regulators, and other health professionals. Results of this work indicated the need for a new nursing professional, the Clinical Nurse Leader (CNL®), who could effectively coordinate, manage, and evaluate care for groups of patients in complex health care systems (Long, 2004). The CNL was to be a lateral integrator for the patient care

119

unit. Lateral integration is the integration of care provided by multiple interdependent and independent disciplines across the continuum of a patient admission or experience (Tornabeni, 2006). The CNL curriculum prepares nurses for clinical leadership and skills in outcomes-based practice. This chapter will outline how to set up a CNL program, develop courses, and establish preceptor partnership.

CNL PROGRAM DEVELOPMENT

Essential ingredients antecedent to successful CNL program development include (a) strong collaborative working relationships between the partnering academic and practice institutions, (b) active engagement of faculty and clinician "champions" of the CNL initiative, (c) presentation of a strong business case for the program and the role, (d) documented support for the resources necessary to implement the program, and (e) documented support for the implementation of the CNL role in the practice environment. Once these fundamental issues are addressed, the academic–practice partnership is well poised to move forward with CNL program development and subsequent role implementation. The key elements of CNL program development to be discussed in this section include resources for program development, adaptation of curriculum, and educational preparation of the CNL.

The most important document guiding the development of a CNL curriculum is AACN's *White Paper on the Education and Role of the Clinical Nurse Leader*™, first drafted in 2003 and then accepted in final form in 2007. This document integrates the graduate level as well as professional entry requirements for CNL curricula and role implementation. As a master's program in nursing, AACN's *The Essentials of Master's Education for Advanced Practice Nursing* (1996) also guides graduate core MSN curriculum. Specific guidance for the CNL curriculum is further explicated in AACN's *Preparing Graduates for Practice as a Clinical Nurse Leader*ˢᵐ *Draft Curriculum Framework* (2006b). AACN has approved five educational models as the starting point for the development of programs to prepare CNLs: BSN-CNL, RN-CNL, second degree students-CNL (AACN, 2007a), Model-B master's degree program for BSN graduates that includes a post-BSN residency that awards master's credit, and a Model-E post-master's certificate program designed for individuals with a master's degree in nursing in another area of study.

Adaptation and/or development of a new curriculum proceeds according to established faculty governance structures and processes within the institution. For new degree programs, additional guidance and preliminary approval by the state board of nursing (for new entry programs), state council of higher education, and the Commission on Collegiate Nursing Education (CCNE) are also necessary. Programs seeking to adapt existing master's curricula into a CNL program of study must also advise CCNE of the change in programming.

Formal curriculum development can be guided by AACN's *CNL*ˢᵐ *Curriculum Framework for Client-Centered Health Care* (Figure 9.1) and/or conceptual models set forth by health care organizations and schools of nursing for development of CNL programs. For example *The Clinical Nurse Leader Conceptual Framework* is based on transition theory and the symptoms management model (Maag, Buccheri, Capella, & Jennings, 2006).

Resources for CNL curriculum development abound and are readily available through the AACN Web site at http://www.aacn.nche. edu/CNL/tkmats.htm. This Web site contains a tool kit replete with documents and resources assimilated for partnerships seeking to develop or expand CNL programs, and the tool kit materials, organized according to Kotter's eight stages of change (Kotter, 1995), are constantly updated.

Essential components of CNL educational preparation identified by the AACN (AACN, 2007b) include fundamental liberal arts education as well as professional values, core nursing knowledge, CNL core competencies, and CNL role development. The CNL curriculum expectations are depicted in Table 9.1.

The post-baccalaureate aspects of CNL education are intended to consist of a 12- to 15-month full-time course of study leading to the advanced generalist master's degree. The final CNL practicum immerses the student in the CNL role. Each student completes at least 300 clinical contact hours enacting the CNL role under the guidance and preceptorship of a master's-prepared clinician who is functioning in a CNL role (or aspect of the CNL role). Aspects of preceptorships and preceptor development are discussed later in this chapter, but from a curriculum development standpoint the AACN provides excellent guidance about the construction of the CNL clinical experiences in the document, *AACN End-of-Program Competencies and Required Clinical Experiences for the Clinical Nurse Leader* (2006a).

<u>Nursing Leadership</u>

I. Horizontal Leadership
II. Effective Use of Self
III. Advocacy
IV. Conceptual Analysis of the CNL Role
V. Lateral Integration of Care

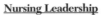

<u>Clinical Outcomes Management</u> ←————→ **<u>Care Environment Management</u>**

I. Illness/Disease Management
  - Care management
  - Client outcomes
  - Builds on and expands the baccalaureate foundation in:
    1. Pharmacology
    2. Physiology/ pathophysiology
    3. Health Assessment

II. Knowledge Management
  - Epidemiology
  - Biostatistics
  - Measurement of client outcomes

III. Health Promotion and Disease Reduction/Prevention Management
  - Risk assessment
  - Health literacy
  - Health education and counseling

IV. Evidence-Based Practice
  - Clinical decision making
  - Critical thinking
  - Problem identification
  - Outcome measurement

I. Team Coordination
  - Delegation
  - Supervision
  - Interdisciplinary care
  - Group process
  - Handling difficult people
  - Conflict resolution

II. Health Care Finance/Economics
  - Medicare and Medicaid/ Reimbursement
  - Resource allocation
  - Health Care technologies
  - Health Care Finance & Socioeconomic Principles

III. Health Care Systems & Organizations
  - Unit level health care delivery/Microsystems of care
  - Complexity theory
  - Managing change theories

IV. Health Care Policy
V. Quality Management/Risk Reduction/Patient Safety
VI. Informatics

Major threads integrated throughout curriculum

I. Critical thinking/Clinical decision making
II. Communication
III. Ethics
IV. Human diversity/cultural competence
V. Global health care
VI. Professional development in the CNL role
VII. Accountability
VIII. Assessment
IX. Nursing technology and resource management
X. Professional values, including social justice

Figure 9.1 CNL curriculum framework for client-centered health care.

From *Preparing Graduates for Practice as a Clinical Nurse Leader*sm *Draft Curriculum Framework*, by AACN, 2006. Retrieved December 15, 2007, from http://www.aacn.nche. edu/CNL/pdf/curricfrmwrk.pdf. Printed with permission.

Table 9.1

CORE COMPETENCY AND ROLE COMPONENTS

1. Liberal arts and sciences background
2. Undergraduate or graduate level coursework in:

   a. Anatomy and physiology

   b. Microbiology

   c. Epidemiology

   d. Statistics

   e. Health care policy

3. Graduate level advancement of the undergraduate foundation in:

   a. Health assessment

   b. Pharmacology

   c. Pathophysiology

4. Institute of Medicine's health professions core competencies:

   a. Quality improvement

   b. Interdisciplinary team care

   c. Patient-centered care

   d. Evidence-based practice

   e. Informatics utilization

5. Clinical contact hours

   a. 400–500 clinical hours total

   b. Minimum of 300 CNL® role immersion clinical hours

COURSE DEVELOPMENT

The AACN task forces on Education and Regulation concluded that the CNL needs specialized knowledge in horizontal leadership, management of care, and care environment management (AACN, 2007b). The CNL curriculum should be developed as a joint venture between practice and education partners. For schools of nursing (SON) this translated into the adaptation of existing master's degree courses and the development of new courses.

Because several national reports were the background for the development of the CNL role (AACN, 2007b; Bartels & Bednash, 2005), the CNL curriculum and courses need to incorporate components of these reports. Specifically, two reports from the IOM were instrumental in the curriculum development: *Crossing the Quality Chasm* (IOM, 2001) and *Health Professions Education: A Bridge to Quality* (IOM, 2003). The Quality Chasm report calls for improvements in six dimensions of health care performance: (a) safety such that patients are as safe in the health care system as they are in their own homes; (b) effectiveness in which care is matched to best science in order to avoid overuse and underuse of effective care; (c) patient-centered care such that a patient's choices, culture, social context, and specific needs are respected; (d) timeliness so that health care performance strives to reduce waiting time and delays for both patients and health care professionals; (e) efficiency such that waste in supplies, equipment, space, capital, and ideas are reduced with a subsequent reduction in cost; and (f) equity in which health care will strive to close racial and ethnic gaps in health status (IOM, 2001).

One of the quality report architects, Donald Berwick, further describes how the report's underlying framework consists of four levels: level A, patient experience; level B, microsystem, which is a unit with a care team; level C, the organization that houses the microsystem; and level D, environment such as policy, payment, regulation, and accreditation. As one moves through the levels, the distance from the patient increases. While changes should happen at all levels, the microsystem is especially important as this "is where the 'quality' experience by the patient is made or lost" (Berwick, 2002, p. 84). The AACN envisioned the CNL as the team leader at the microsystem level, but in order to be an effective team leader the CNL needs knowledge about both the whole system and how to be an efficient team leader (AACN, 2007b).

The second IOM report states that health care professionals need educational practice in the system described in the quality chasm report. In such a system, all graduates have to demonstrate achievement in five health professions core competencies: (a) quality improvement; (b) interdisciplinary team care; (c) patient-centered care; (d) evidence-based practice; and (e) utilization of informatics (IOM, 2003). All of these components are included in the CNL curriculum, so that the CNL can act as a lateral integrator of care, a patient advocate over the many components of the continuum of care, and an information manager to the multiple disciplines involved in care (Harris, Tornabeni, & Walters, 2006).

So how do these reports and their conclusions translate into the CNL curriculum? AACN together with nurse leaders (AACN, 2007b; Bartels, 2005; Tornabeni, 2006) stress that the curriculum has to include the following components shown in Exhibit 9.1.

Exhibit 9.1

ESSENTIAL CNL CURRICULUM COMPONENTS

1. Nursing leadership, that is, how to effectively work with others to improve quality.

2. Providing and managing care, that is, how to coordinate the health care team and maximize the abilities of the nurse providing direct patient care.

3. Care environment management, that is, how to use knowledge about team coordination and strategies for making change at the microsystem level.

4. Clinical outcomes management, that is, how to use knowledge from the biological sciences for illness/disease management.

5. Health promotion/risk reduction for individuals and populations, that is, how to use knowledge management to understand cause-and-effect relationships, including the ways that culture, ethnicity, and socioeconomic variations affect health status and response to health care.

6. Evidence-based practice, that is, how to use critical thinking and analysis of research findings to plan evidence-based interventions.

7. Quality, safety, and risk management, that is, how to anticipate and avoid risks to patient safety, for example using Root Cause Analysis, Failure Mode Effects Analysis, and other tools for quality improvement.

8. Health care technologies such as information technology (IT) systems and databases, that is, how to utilize databases to establish trends in order to improve plans of care.

9. Health care systems and organizations, that is, how to use systems theory and complexity theory to deliver microsystem care, suggest policy changes in the organization, and understand state/national health care policy.

10. Health care finance and regulation, that is, how to use knowledge and understanding of the cost of care to enhance efficiency with which care is delivered.

Note: From *White Paper on the Education and Role of the Clinical Nurse Leader*™, by AACN, February 2007. Retrieved December 15, 2007, from http://www.aacn.nche.edu/Publications/WhitePapers/ClinicalNurseLeader07.pdfAACN. Adapted with permission.

One could argue that some of these subjects are already taught in undergraduate and graduate nursing programs; therefore a closer examination of the CNL and other nursing education curricula is warranted.

CNL and Other Nursing Curricula

It has been suggested that the role of the CNL is a combination of a staff nurse with an undergraduate degree and other advanced nursing roles such as clinical nurse specialist (CNS), nurse practitioner (NP), case manager, and nurse manager (Erickson & Ditomassi, 2005). However, in the American Organization of Nurse Executive's Guiding Principles, a comparison of the CNL role and the baccalaureate-level nurse clearly states that the CNL has competencies and knowledge of a graduate nurse (Haase-Herrick & Herrin, 2007). The CNL generally has a more robust knowledge of health care financing and quality, safety, and statistical processes. The CNL role also differs from the advanced practice role of the NP and CNS as the CNL is a generalist and the CNS and NP are specialists. One hospital employed NPs in the CNL role and found that working as a CNL did not allow the NP to use her advanced practice direct patient care skills (Bowcutt, Wall, & Goolsby, 2006). Another advanced practice role that overlaps with the CNL is that of a case manager. However, case management is different, as the nurse case manager is assigned to a specific patient or group of patients and generally does not oversee care delivery at the clinical point of care (Begun, Hamilton, Tornabeni, & White, 2006). In contrast, the CNL is assigned to a nursing unit to oversee and deliver direct patient care. The CNL role also includes management components (Ott, Haase-Herrick, & Harris, 2006). In order to be an effective lateral integrator and team leader the CNL needs knowledge about management principles, but the CNL does not have the management responsibility of overseeing administration of nursing unit(s).

When considering what courses are needed in a CNL curriculum, it is clear that some CNL classes do overlap with other advanced degree curricula. For example, classes in pathophysiology, pharmacology, epidemiology, evidence-based practice, and health policy are not specific to a CNL program. However due to the nature of the CNL role, classes in leadership development and care environment management are unique to the CNL program. The inclusion of CNL-specific course work requires having faculty who are prepared to teach in areas not typically included in graduate nursing programs. For example, the leadership classes rely heavily on the development and evaluation of the individual student's leadership skills, and the care environment management classes emphasize understanding of systems and transforming that understanding to the microsystem level. Both of these class series require that schools of nursing look critically at the skills of their faculty and either educate faculty in these content areas or "borrow" faculty or classes from other departments, such as psychology, sociology, health administration, public health, and health care economics.

Leadership Development and Care Environment Management

Educating a CNL requires greater attention to the context and development of leadership skills (Bartels, 2005). Courses in leadership skills and interpersonal development should be included in any CNL curriculum. In addition, the CNL courses in care environment management teach the student how to implement or change system processes both at the microsystem and organization level. Conflict resolution, risk taking, and critical analysis of evidence for quality improvements, as well as how to access data and use IT systems are other aspects covered in care environment management classes (AACN, 2007b).

Through these courses the CNLs develop well-honed skills in communication, critical thinking, and interaction modalities. They are taught how to access, evaluate, and disseminate knowledge at the system level. Further, the courses teach the CNL to justify clinical actions based on evidence, and then incorporate evidence into practice and the education of others. Students learn how to challenge current policies and procedures and practice environments using change theory and the theory of diffusion of dissemination. The CNLs also acquire knowledge and understanding of information systems and standardized languages. These skills are used to evaluate and improve care of the client and to compare outcomes with standards (Bartels, 2005).

Furthermore, the courses' content prepares the CNL to make true integration possible across provider settings and experiment with new models of care delivery driven by changing consumer needs while also considering the fiscal soundness of the system (Haase-Herrick, 2005). The CNL acquires a functional applied understanding of basic business skills and organizational theory that prepares them for the fiscal context in which they are practicing, enabling them to identify the high-cost/high-volume activities associated with care delivery. The knowledge and skills of the CNL make them able to play a role in policy formation at the systems level, as well as how to influence policies for clinical populations and whole communities that are suffering health disparities (Bartels, 2005).

In summary, a well-thought-out curriculum can use existing graduate nursing programs in conjunction with the development of courses in leadership and care environment management. Because the CNLs are evaluated in how they apply the course concepts in clinical practice, the practice partnership between practice sites and schools of nursing is vital for a successful CNL curriculum. The next section describes how preceptor partnerships are developed.

PRECEPTOR PARTNERSHIPS

CNL education is a joint venture between practice and education. The innovation that supports CNL education and is highly anticipated in program graduates is enhanced by clinical preceptorships. Clinical education that is guided and overseen by preceptors provides CNL students with support during their clinical learning, as they encounter new experiences, try on new skills, and have opportunities to experience the reality of clinical practice. Preceptorships are based on the assumption that a consistent one-to-one relationship provides opportunities for socialization into practice and bridges the gap between theory and practice. The theory-practice gap is the discrepancy between what students are taught in the classroom (the theoretic aspects of nursing) and what they experience in clinical placement (Corlett, 2000). The components important for successful preceptor partnerships to be discussed in this section are role modeling, creating an open forum for mutual learning, qualities of a good preceptor, and preceptor support.

Role Modeling

A clinical preceptor is an experienced nurse who assumes the role of clinical teacher for a student. Preceptor–student dyads serve to socialize students into professional nursing through access to and relationship with excellent role models. The preceptorship connection provides a strong model for the student to observe and emulate. The importance of a positive attitude and behavior when acting as a role model is undeniable to a successful preceptorship (Firtko, Stewart, & Knox, 2005). In addition to role modeling, Myrick and Yonge (2004) identify three additional roles of the preceptor: facilitation, guidance, and prioritization. Facilitation occurs when preceptors support learners rather than direct or teach. Guidance is related to facilitation and involves the preceptor guiding the student in their practice. Prioritization is helping the student plan and evaluate care for a group of patients.

Creating an Open Forum for Mutual Learning

The preceptor partnership needs to be in an environment that fosters mutual learning. For critical thinking to occur, students need to feel a sense of security in putting forth their ideas and points of view. Students also need to be able to trust their preceptors' acceptance and support of their questioning. They need to be able to believe that independence of thought is truly valued and that the relationship is not about pleasing the preceptor. Thus, the environment most effective in enhancing critical thinking is one that reflects support; is devoid of threat; and fosters openness, inquiry, and trust (Myrick, 2002). Preceptor–student dyads are key to promoting critical thinking. Myrick (2002) found that the one-to-one relationship figured prominently in the enhancement of students' critical thinking. Critical thinking prepares students to reason and to make sound patient care judgments. It equips students with the ability to scrutinize relevant nursing interventions, examine the consequences of decisions, consider a variety of nursing care perspectives, and evaluate care that is provided. This is an essential issue in CNL clinical education. CNLs are taught to question, to challenge, and to use recent evidence in planning care. CNL preceptors must be sufficiently confident to allow students to challenge practice strategies and pose difficult questions. Preceptors set the tone for the learning climate through their supportive attitudes, by valuing the preceptees, and by their ability to work with them throughout the experience (Myrick & Yonge, 2004).

The CNL role may be perceived as a threat to other roles; therefore, the preceptorship enables students to hone their understanding of the CNL vision and goals, to defuse defensiveness, to discuss potential beneficial outcomes, and to promote acceptance. Stanley, Hoiting, Burton, Harris, & Norman (2007) describe staff nurse understanding of the CNL vision and goal as the most significant part of its success. Staff nurses need to understand how the CNL can reduce care fragmentation, elevate nursing practice, and enable staff nurses to expand their practice while remaining at the bedside. Preceptorships can foster this understanding. The CNL role focuses on understanding the interdependency of all disciplines providing care. It is essential, therefore, that team relationships be fostered. Preceptors may do this by facilitating introductions to all members of the team, by assuring that the student's name is included with staff assignments on the daily assignment sheet or greaseboard, and by inviting the student to join the staff at lunch and breaks.

The practical aspects of designing clinical experiences with preceptors include facilitating maximal schedule flexibility. This may be achieved by block scheduling classes to promote student availability to work the preceptor's schedule. This approach also strengthens student understanding of clinical practice reality through regular opportunities to work day, evening, night, and weekend shifts. Students learn to gather needed patient and clinical information during the clinical day. This is facilitated by ready access to electronic resources. Students and preceptors need mechanisms to contact clinical faculty whenever the student is in the clinical setting. Faculty monitor student progress through participation in clinical rounds to the practice areas, students' participation in conferences, student/preceptor/faculty conferences, and students' written assignments.

Qualities of a Good Preceptor

Clinical preceptors need to be selected carefully. Not all exemplary clinicians are good clinical teachers. Every preceptor needs certain key qualities: clinical expertise, organizational skills, teaching talent, patience, leadership, and the desire to be a preceptor (Zwerneman & Flanders, 2006). A willingness to work together, gaining mutual understanding, and having a sense of humor are also essential to collaborative efforts (Palmer, Cox, Callister, Johnson, & Matsumara, 2005). For CNL students, preceptors must also be prepared at the Bachelor of Science in Nursing (BSN) level or higher, enjoy working with students, possess a positive attitude toward teaching and learning, be open to innovative approaches, have excellent interpersonal skills and excellent communication skills, and buy in to the CNL role. The role and qualities of the preceptor are outlined in Table 9.2.

Preceptor Support

There are challenges to the preceptor–student relationship and model. At a fundamental level, the model involves matching two strangers for

Table 9.2

CNL FACT PRECEPTOR EXPECTATIONS

1. Review all medications.
2. Supervise all clinical skills.
3. Foster critical thinking by questioning students on the rationale for nursing and medical interventions.
4. Immerse and engage students in clinical practice experiences, integrating them into the practice setting.
5. Negotiate clinical learning objectives prior to each clinical experience.
6. Assist in the assessment of student performance.

    a. Give in-the-moment verbal feedback.

    b. Complete written mid-term and final evaluations.

    c. Inform clinical faculty of student progress, issues, concerns.
7. Assist the student to revise his/her objectives for the clinical experiences.

    a. Use objectives to plan clinical experiences.

    b. Assist student and clinical faculty in planning additional clinical experiences to meet student needs and enhance learning.

---

an important and essential experience. It is within a challenging work environment that these two strangers must learn to accommodate one another in a professional capacity (Yonge, Myrick, & Haase, 2002). Precepting is much more than asking a student to "shadow" or follow the nurse. Precepting requires added time and energy, which can be a source of stress in the workplace for nurses who already feel overburdened with their current workloads (Hautala, Saylor, & O'Leary-Kelly, 2007). There are real time constraints that may require the preceptor to prioritize between focusing on providing care to the patient or teaching the student.

Preceptors need ongoing support. This support may be provided by clinical faculty, course professors, and mentors such as advanced practice nurses, educators, managers, and experienced preceptors (Zwerneman & Flanders, 2006). They need support in developing teaching skills, handling the day-to-day demands, handling the variety of learning styles, and other challenging teaching/learning situations. Preceptors need to be taught strategies to deal with conflict effectively, accept different learning styles, and create win-win situations (Speers, Strzyzewski, & Ziolkowski, 2004). Faculty should not underestimate the importance of a nurturing and supportive faculty–preceptor relationship. Preceptors appreciate formal evaluation of how they are doing, and site visits by faculty help provide a realistic view of students' performance and a forum for mutual feedback. Clinical site visits also allow faculty and preceptors an opportunity for face-to-face acknowledgement of preceptor contribution and support for the preceptor role (Campbell & Hawkins, 2007). An area that preceptors need guidance is in providing evaluative feedback. Preceptors are often reluctant to provide negative feedback that may negatively influence the student's grade or progression through the program. Preceptors must also recognize that they can never be consistently aware of their own actions and cognizant of the impact those actions have on others. Preceptors must remind themselves of the intrinsic power they possess with regard to the evaluative role (Myrick & Yonge, 2004).

To promote preceptor retention and recruitment, preceptors must be recognized and rewarded for their contributions to student education. Rewards acknowledge the essential role of the preceptor, and not all rewards need to be monetary. Serving as preceptor will likely contribute to the advancement of the nurse. Additional rewards may include adjunct clinical faculty status, certificate of recognition, dinner/luncheon, continuing education talks, verification of hours toward certification, letter of thanks from the school, outstanding preceptor award, participation in projects or research, faculty who provide in-services, and faculty who edit manuscripts (Campbell & Hawkins, 2007). Preceptors have the ability to create a learning environment that fosters human potential, professional development, and mutual understanding (Palmer et al., 2005). Precepting is an art that must be crafted over time, based on knowledge, skill, and experience. Both students and preceptors benefit from a successful (preceptor) partnership (see Table 9.3).

SUMMARY AND FUTURE DIRECTIONS

In summary, a carefully developed CNL program will include a strong practice partnership and a curriculum that prepares the CNL to be certified as such and to practice as a lateral integrator in the patient care unit engaged in outcome-based practice and quality improvement strategies. In April 2007, 130 CNLs had graduated from the about 90 pilot programs in the country (Stringer, 2007). The CNL programs are dispersed across the country with the first 76 programs located in 37 states and one territory (Stanhope & Turner, 2006). The practice-partnerships formed suggest that the CNL program can be developed in many settings; for example, most schools were not located in academic health centers (66%) and most practice sites did not have Magnet accreditation (75%).

One can question whether we need another nursing program (Grindel, 2005; National Association of Clinical Nurse Specialists, 2004). However, with the CNL program we might attract students that would not otherwise have considered a nursing career for second degree programs or graduate nursing education. The CNLs that enter through the second degree programs often have different expectations and ask other

Table 9.3

OUTCOMES FOR STUDENTS AND PRECEPTORS

STUDENT OUTCOMES

- Smooth transition to clinical environment
- Increased clinical experiences
- Improved communication
- Improved leadership
- Increased confidence
- Improved organizational and clinical proficiency
- Real-world expectations
- Validation of chosen profession

PRECEPTORS OUTCOMES

- Stimulate own professional growth
- Personal satisfaction
- Increased job satisfaction
- Decreased staff turnover

questions than the "regular" graduate nursing student. Many of these CNL students come from fields other than health care, and many have a wealth of knowledge and experience that influence their learning and professional development within the health care system. With the growing nursing shortage should we not welcome anybody that is willing and able to become a nurse? Nursing programs that produce high quality bedside leaders and clinicians should be a welcome addition to the ever-increasing complexities of our health care system. Moreover, early pilot studies suggest that implementation of the CNL role improves patient outcomes such as falls, pressure ulcers, nosocomial infections, and patient satisfaction; nurse outcomes such as turnover rates, collaboration, and satisfaction; and administrative outcomes such as length of stay and decreased use of travel nurses (Hartranft, Garcia, & Adams, 2007; Smith & Dabbs, 2007; Smith, Manfredi, Drummond-Huth, Hagos, & Moore, 2006; Stanley et al., 2007).

Proponents of the CNL program posit that this is a step to adequately prepare the next generation of nurses to participate as full partners in shaping the future and improving patient care outcomes. Another bold step would be to include students from other health care fields in part of the CNL curriculum. As was mentioned earlier, some unique CNL courses include competencies such as quality improvement, interdisciplinary team care, patient-centered care, evidence-based practice, and utilization of informatics that IOM (2003) has deemed important for all health care graduates. This would produce health care graduates that are skilled in interdisciplinary teamwork before they enter the health care field as independent practitioners.

REFERENCES

American Association of Colleges of Nursing. (1996). *The essentials of master's education for advanced practice nursing.* Retrieved December 15, 2007, from http://www.aacn.nche.edu/Education/pdf/MasEssentials96.pdf

American Association of Colleges of Nursing. (2006a, May). *AACN end-of-program competencies and required clinical experiences for the Clinical Nurse Leader.* Retrieved December 15, 2007, from http://www.aacn.nche.edu/CNL/pdf/EndComps grid.pdf

American Association of Colleges of Nursing. (2006b). *Preparing graduates for practice as a Clinical Nurse Leader^sm draft curriculum framework.* Retrieved December 15, 2007, from http://www.aacn.nche.edu/CNL/pdf/curricfrmwrk.pdf

American Association of Colleges of Nursing. (2007a, November). *Clinical Nurse Leader (CNL) frequently asked questions.* Retrieved December 15, 2007, from http://www.aacn.nche.edu/CNL/pdf/CNLFAQ.pdf

American Association of Colleges of Nursing. (2007b, February). *White paper on the education and role of the Clinical Nurse Leader.*™ Retrieved December 15, 2007, from http://www.aacn.nche.edu/Publications/WhitePapers/ClinicalNurseLeader07.pdf

Bartels, J. E. (2005). Educating nurses for the 21st century. *Nursing & Health Sciences, 7,* 221–225.

Bartels, J. E., & Bednash, G. (2005). Answering the call for quality nursing care and patient safety. *Nursing Administration Quarterly, 29*(1), 5–13.

Begun, J. W., Hamilton, J. A., Tornabeni, J., & White, K. R. (2006). Opportunities for improving patient care through lateral integration: The Clinical Nurse Leader. *Journal of Healthcare Management, 51,* 19–25.

Berwick, D. (2002). A user's manual for the IOM's quality chasm report. *Health Affairs, 21*(3), 80–90.

Bowcutt, M., Wall, J., & Goolsby, M. J. (2006). The Clinical Nurse Leader: Promoting patient-centered outcomes. *Nursing Administration Quarterly, 30,* 156–161.

Campbell, S. H., & Hawkins, J. W. (2007). Preceptor rewards: How to say thank you for mentoring the next generation of nurse practitioners. *Journal of the American Academy of Nurse Practitioners, 19,* 24–29.

Corlett, J. (2000). The perceptions of nurse teachers, student nurses and preceptors of the theory-practice gap in nurse education. *Nurse Education Today, 20,* 499–505.

Erickson, J. I., & Ditomassi, M. (2005). The Clinical Nurse Leader: New in name only. *Journal of Nursing Education, 44,* 99–100.

Firtko, A., Stewart, R., & Knox, N. (2005). Understanding mentoring and preceptorship: Clarifying the quagmire. *Contemporary Nurse, 19,* 32.

Grindel, C. (2005). From AMSN: AACN presents the clinical nurse leader and the doctor in nursing practice roles: A benefit or a misfortune? *MEDSURG Nursing, 14*(4), 209–210.

Haase-Herrick, K. S. (2005). The opportunities of stewardship. *Nursing Administration Quarterly, 29,* 115–118.

Haase-Herrick, K. S., & Herrin, D. M. (2007). The American Organization of Nurse Executives' guiding principles and American Association of Colleges of Nursing's Clinical Nurse Leader: A lesson in synergy. *Journal of Nursing Administration, 37,* 55–60.

Harris, J. L., Tornabeni, J., & Walters, S. E. (2006). The Clinical Nurse Leader: A valued member of the healthcare team. *Journal of Nursing Administration, 36,* 446–449.

Hartranft, S. R., Garcia, T., & Adam, N. (2007). Realizing the anticipated effects of the Clinical Nurse Leader. *Journal of Nursing Administration, 37,* 261–263.

Hautala, K. T., Saylor, C. R., & O'Leary-Kelly, C. (2007). Nurses' perceptions of stress and support in the preceptor role. *Journal for Nurses in Staff Development, 23,* 64–70.

Institute of Medicine (IOM). (2001). *Crossing the quality chasm.* Washington, DC: National Academy Press.

Institute of Medicine (IOM). (2003). *Health professions education: A bridge to quality.* Washington, DC: National Academy Press.

Kotter, J. P. (1995). Leading change: Why transformation efforts fail. *Harvard Business Review, 75*(2), 59–67.

Long, K. A. (2004). Preparing nurses for the 21st century: Reenvisioning nursing education and practice. *Journal of Professional Nursing, 20,* 82–88.

Maag, M. M., Buccheri, R., Capella, E., & Jennings, D. L. (2006). A conceptual framework for a Clinical Nurse Leader program. *Journal of Professional Nursing, 22,* 367–372.

Myrick, F. (2002). Preceptorship and critical thinking in nursing education. *Journal of Nursing Education, 41,* 154–163.

Myrick, F., & Yonge, O. (2004). Enhancing critical thinking in the preceptorship experience in nursing education. *Journal of Advanced Nursing, 459,* 371–380.

National Association of Clinical Nurse Specialists. (2004, March). *NACNS position statement on the Clinical Nurse Leader.* Retrieved January 2, 2007, from http://www.nacns.org/positionstatement.pdf

Ott, K. M., Haase-Herrick, K., & Harris, J. (2006, March). *American Association of Colleges of Nursing working statement comparing the Clinical Nurse Leader*sm *and nurse manager roles: Similarities, differences and complementarities.* Retrieved December 15, 2007, from http://www.aacn.nche.edu/CNL/pdf/tk/roles3–06.pdf

Palmer, S. P., Cox, A. H., Callister, L. C., Johnson, V., & Matsumara, G. (2005). Nursing education and service collaboration: Making a difference in the clinical learning environment. *The Journal of Continuing Education in Nursing, 36*(6), 271–276.

Radzyminski, S. (2005). Advances in graduate nursing education: Beyond the advanced practice nurse. *Journal of Professional Nursing, 21,* 119–125.

Smith, D. S., & Dabbs, M. T. (2007). Transforming the care delivery model in preparation for the Clinical Nurse Leader. *Journal of Nursing Administration, 37,* 157–160.

Smith, S. L., Manfredi, T., Drummond-Huth, B., Hagos, O. & Moore, P. (2006). Application of the Clinical Nurse Leader role in an acute care delivery model. *Journal of Nursing Administration, 36,* 29–33.

Speers, A. T., Strzyzewski, N., & Ziolkowski, L. D. (2004). Preceptor preparation: An investment in the future. *Journal for Nurses in Staff Development, 20*(3), 127–133.

Stanhope, M., & Turner, L. (2006). Diffusion of the Clinical Nurse Leader innovation. *Journal of Nursing Administration, 36,* 385–389.

Stanley, J. M., Hoiting, T., Burton, D., Harris, J., & Norman, L. (2007). Implementing innovation through education-practice partnerships. *Nursing Outlook, 55,* 67–73.

Stringer, H. (2007). Clinical Nurse Leader: New role focuses on big picture. *NurseWeek California, 20*(8), 10–12.

Tornabeni, J. (2006). The evolution of a revolution in nursing. *Journal of Nursing Administration, 36,* 3–6.

Yonge, O., Myrick, F., & Haase, M. (2002). Student nurse stress in the preceptorship experience. *Nurse Educator, 27*(2), 84–88.

Zwerneman, K., & Flanders, S. (2006). Do you want to be a preceptor? *American Nurse Today, 1*(11), 35–36.

10

Credentialing, Licensure, and Certification Considerations

VICTORIA A. WEILL, JUNE A. TRESTON, AND ANN L. O'SULLIVAN

Credentialing is an important and essential aspect of clinical practice. Scope and standards of practice are matched with specific levels of education and clinical preparation to credential nurses. This process protects the public and ensures safety and quality of care. The advent of the Doctor of Nursing Practice (DNP) and the Clinical Nurse Leader (CNL®) represent change that may impact credentialing, licensure, and certification.

Nurses holding advanced degrees are credentialed through several entities that are each essential to practice. This chapter will explore three aspects of the credentialing process. The first is credentialing by state government through licensure. Licensure or other types of state recognition allow qualified candidates to practice with an extended scope of practice in a focused population. The second type of credentialing is through certification. Professional certifying organizations, such as the American Nurse Credentialing Center (ANCC), offer specialty exams that recognize nurses' advanced knowledge and expertise. The final form of credentialing that will be explored is through employer institutions. Such credentialing is mandated by national agencies such as the Joint Commission (TJC) and includes verification of licensure, national and state certification, and a detailed ongoing review of practice and criminal history.

This chapter will explore important practice questions related to credentialing. The following will be addressed:

- In the future, will every advanced practice registered nurse (APRN) have a second nursing license?
- Will all nurse practitioners be required to earn a DNP?
- Will the National Council of State Boards of Nursing (NCSBN) develop a licensure examination to test the entry-level competence of APRNs?
- Will national specialty exams thrive in the future?

HISTORICAL PERSPECTIVES ON CREDENTIALING, LICENSING, AND CERTIFICATION

Credentialing History

Credentialing is "a process . . . encompassing a variety of mechanisms that share a set of common goals: to ensure quality, competency and accountability and to achieve recognition." (McGivern, Sullivan-Marx, & Mezey, 2003, p. 3). It is an umbrella term that encompasses concepts such as licensure, certification, and the credentialing of employees by institutions or insurance plans.

In 1976, the American Nurses Association (ANA) appointed a study committee to investigate and suggest improvements for the credentialing system that included accreditation, certification, and licensure. Seventy agencies concerned with credentialing in nursing convened. Out of this work group came the development of some principles of credentialing, but more important was the recommendation that a center was needed to conduct nursing credentialing. This was the birth of the American Nurses Credentialing Center (ANA, 1979).

While the levels of credentialing used for regulation can be applied to any profession, examination of these levels (National Council of State Boards of Nursing [NCSBN], 1993) provides a good sense of how the nursing profession has developed. The least restrictive type of regulation is designation/recognition. The board does not investigate a nurse's competence or restrict their practice; it simply recognizes an individual's special qualifications. The next level is registration. The names of nurses are simply listed on an official state board of nursing (SBON) roster. Competence is not investigated, and usually scope of practice is

not delineated. Certification is the third level. There is often some confusion because the term *certification* is used both by the professional
organization and the regulatory bodies. While a SBON sometimes uses
professional certification as an equivalent for regulatory certification or
licensure, in the legal sense, certification refers to APRNs who have met
certain stipulations and are "certified." Licensure is the fourth level and
usually includes adherence to a unique scope of practice. A high level of
accountably is expected in order to protect the public health and safety.

Regulation/Licensure History

Early developments in the U.S. history of licensing of health care providers have had a significant impact on APRNs. By the early 1900s, physicians were the first licensed. Their comprehensive medical practice
acts created a near monopoly on the "entire human condition" and any
actions directed at "health or sickness" became their sole responsibility.
These ubiquitous medical practice acts continue to remain on the books
in almost every state. Every time nursing (or another profession) wants
to expand its scope of practice a turf battle ensues because medicine
perceives this as an infringement of its domain (Safriet, 2002).

Bullough (1982) describes the history of nurse practice law occurring in three phases. The first phase began in 1903 when North Carolina passed the first licensure law defining the registered nurse. These
registered nurses could be distinguished because they had completed a
formal program and had passed a state board examination. The second
phase occurred with legislation in New York in 1938, which limited nursing functions to nurses. To do this, scope of practice statements had to
be developed to delineate what constituted a nursing function. In 1955
the ANA defined the professional practice of the registered nurse. One
key phrase served to be especially problematic for APRNs: "The forego-
ing shall not be deemed to include any acts of diagnosis or prescription
of therapeutic or corrective measures" (ANA, 1955). The exclusion of diagnosis and treatment would directly impact APRNs. A number of states
used the ANA's definition of nursing in their laws. In the ensuing years,
formal nurse practitioner (NP) programs were developed, and the first
NPs graduated from the University of Colorado's pediatric nurse practitioner program in 1965 (McAtee & Silver, 1974). Increasing numbers of
nurses were performing in expanded roles; this included the diagnosis
and treatment of patients. Numerous states had to rewrite their practice acts to accommodate all of the expanded functions of the advanced

practice nurse. In 1971, through changes in their nurse practice act, Idaho was the first state to formally recognize advanced practice nursing as different from that provided by RNs (phase 3). This was followed by changes to New York's practice act, in 1972, allowing diagnosis and treatment by nurse practitioners.

A fourth licensing phase began in the early 1990s when NCSBN proposed a second license to regulate APRNs (Porcher, 2003). APRNs were providing complex care requiring advanced knowledge, independent decision making, and autonomy. Unlike the RN level, which had a single National Council Licensure Examination (NCLEX) to ensure the achievement of baseline knowledge for all test takers, there was tremendous diversity in educational programs, requirements of certifying bodies, and numbers of certification exams at the APRN level. For example, there were nurses functioning in advanced practice roles that trained in certificate programs of variable length who had not received advanced graduate education. This variability created confusion.

The NCSBN worried that this unevenness would impact the public's health and safety. They proposed a second license as a means of protecting the public by defining a unique expanded scope of practice and providing legal authority to advanced practice nurses. A second license would ensure a minimum set of competencies, given the various routes of entry into the role. Licensure also assures that complex care will be provided by qualified providers who are held accountable for their practice. Finally, licensure provides a forum for the public to resolve complaints about competency and provides a means for disciplinary action. Others continue to argue that statutory regulation is not necessary. They feel that other professions, for example, law, medicine, and dentistry, initially mandate a license for beginning practitioners, then use professional certification as a mechanism for specialization and a means to demonstrate added expertise. But a nurse's first level of education is not the same for all who enter the profession; thus, a second license documents consistency in all APRN education, protecting both the public and the APRN.

NCSBN questioned whether they should offer an umbrella APRN core exam (like the NCLEX for RNs) that all APRNs (CNPs, CNMs, CRNAs, and CNSs) would take for regulatory purposes. An alternate possibility was to use the certification examinations already in place as one of the steps for licensure. Unfortunately, these certification exams were not originally designed for regulatory purposes. There was a need to ensure that each professional organization's certification process, particularly the examination portion, was adequately rigorous to provide regulatory sufficiency. The task of this evaluation was given to NCCA (National Commission of Certifying Agencies), the certifying body for NOCA (National Organization of Competency Assurance) and the American Board of Nursing Specialties (ABNS). NCSBN was assured that the examinations of the national certifying organizations (such as American Nurses Credentialing Center [ANCC] & Pediatric Nursing Certification Board [PNCB]) were psychometrically sound and legally defensible. The concept of a single core exam for all NPs was laid to rest.

Certification History

Historically, nurses chose voluntary certification as a way to demonstrate expert knowledge and excellence in a specialty area. For some, it was a way to receive professional recognition and advancement. Surprisingly, CRNAs were the first APRNs certified as far back as 1945 (Hanson, 2005). CNMs were certified in 1971 (Dorroh & Kelley, 2005). The first certification exam for nurse practitioners was offered in 1975 by the National Certification Board of Pediatric Nurse Practitioners and Associates (now PNCB) for pediatric nurse practitioners (McLeod, 1995). This was soon followed by exams for a variety of nurses, both APRNs and non-APRNs, offered by ANCC starting in the late 1970. In the early years, significant accompanying materials had to be submitted with the examination application, including documentation such as case studies, nursing philosophies, and information about a nurse's clinical practice setting (Millonig, 1986). The credentialing process gave nurses formal recognition of their expanded role.

Certification changes occurred in the 1990s as the role for NPs expanded beyond the scope of RN practice and some SBONs began to require a second license for this new scope. Certification exams now were used to test minimal-level competency for new graduates. These exams shifted from demonstrating the attainment of excellence in practice to becoming a proxy licensure examination needed to indicate entry-level knowledge.

The National Association of Clinical Nurse Specialists emphasizes that the "essence of CNS [clinical nurse specialist] expertise is embedded in a specialty," with as many as 42 different specialties available (2003). It has been difficult and expensive for individual specialty organizations to create valid exams for small numbers of applicants. To date, state boards of nursing continue to insist on successful exam results to document beginning practice knowledge as a CNS. Philosophical disagreements continue regarding the appropriateness of other mechanisms such as portfolios to demonstrate this same competency for beginning practitioners.

Employer/Institutional Credentialing History

The Joint Commission began around 1910 with a goal of improving hospital care (TJC, 2008). Patients were tracked to determine if a hospital's treatments had been effective, and if not, why not. Over the years, a continuous goal was the quality and safety of clinical care. A component involved monitoring the quality of the medical staff. In 1965, in a pivotal court case, a lawsuit involving a bad medical outcome determined that hospitals have a corporate liability for the quality of the medical staff. Credentialing the provider staff is one way to ensure certain performance standards. Until recently, APRNs in hospitals were not credentialed with the same formal process as the medical staff. Many times they were not evaluated at all, because they were considered to be under the physician's supervision. If Advanced Practice Registered Nurses (APRNs) were reviewed, it was a simple process done by the personnel department (Jones, 2002). This is no longer enough. APRNs' level of responsibility has increased. Meeting TJC standards is also required for hospitals to be eligible for Medicaid and Medicare funding. Today, APRNs working in institutions are being evaluated with the same rigorous credentialing process as the medical staff.

CURRENT TRENDS IN NURSING EDUCATION AND IMPLICATIONS FOR REGULATION

Recently there has been a growth in the development of educational programs to prepare nurses for advanced practice as APRNs. Since the curriculum of these programs varies, students may graduate with different skill sets and knowledge. Variation in educational preparation will impact licensure, certification, and credentialing.

The master's degree remains the foundation of traditional programs preparing APRNs. Broad population content and clinical experience allow graduates to practice in varied settings and care for focused patient groups which span the continuum of health care. To assure that specific content and clinical hours are included, the curriculum of each program is closely monitored through each individual state board of nursing, as well as certifying (such as the ANCC and PNCB); and accrediting (such as the Commission on Collegiate Nursing Education [CCNE] and National League for Nursing Accrediting Commission [NLNAC]) organizations. This is important, as the licensing/certification of graduates is dependent on the successful completion of an approved program. There are several safeguards in place to assure the NCSBN that educational programs meet approved standards.

For example, a Certified Nurse Practitioner (CNP) APRN program's curricula must meet the National Organization of Nurse Practitioner Faculties (NONPF) Core Competencies, the American Association of Colleges of Nursing (AACN) Essentials of Master's Education, or Essentials of Doctoral Education for Advanced Nursing Practice (AACN, 2006) and the National Task Force on Quality NP Education (NTF) evaluation criteria for CNP education programs (NTF, 2008). These documents provide an important structure to ensure that CNP APRNs will receive fundamental knowledge as part of strong educational programs. Each program that prepares APRNs must include the core science content, advanced health/physical assessment, advanced physiology/pathophysiology, and advanced pharmacology. A program must cover all the specific content to be eligible for accreditation by CCNE (the accrediting arm of AACN) or NLNAC (the corresponding division of the National League of Nursing [NLN]). Programs are also reviewed by the certifying organizations, such as the ANCC and PNCB, to ensure that they meet key educational standards. The new APRN Regulatory Model works to eliminate this redundancy of program review. Programs will be reviewed by the national accrediting bodies. Even now a number of certifying entities rely on review by the accrediting bodies.

In order to sit for a national certification organization's examination, an applicant must be a graduate of a recognized program. The American Board of Nursing Specialties (ABNS) and the National Commission for Certifying Agencies (NCCA) are umbrella associations that provide accreditation for the certifying organizations. These groups are responsible for ensuring that consistent national standards are applied when certifying nurses as APRNs. Furthermore, ABNS and NCCA ensure that certifying organizations meet their obligation to construct certifying exams that are reflective of approved APRN curriculum and are psycho-metrically sound and legally defensible.

Accreditation for certifying organizations provides safeguards that have helped the NCSBN feel comfortable in accepting national certi-fication as "partial fulfillment of regulatory requirements for APRNs" (NCSBN, 2002, p. 3) and avoid a need to go to the expense of devel-oping their own exams and processes. This reassurance has helped the NCSBN drop the notion of creating a single core exam for APRNs, simi-lar to the NCLEX for RNs. With statutory recognition of APRNs to be eligible for third-party reimbursement and prescriptive privileges, stan-dards and higher accountability have become even more important to the credentialing process.

A new educational program preparing some APRNs is the DNP. The impact of the DNP versus the traditional research-based PhD on the nursing workforce is currently under debate. A DNP program may pre-pare the graduate for one of the four APRN roles. However, some DNP programs are designed for individuals who already hold a master's de-gree and certification in one of the four APRN roles. These post-master's DNP programs are primarily not designed to prepare new APRNs. The DNP prepares students to become expert nurses, but it may not meet the educational criteria for the four APRN roles. For those individuals already qualified to practice as an APRN, the addition of a DNP will not currently change their licensed scope of practice. It is likely that DNP graduates will advocate for future change in the Nurse Practice Act to reflect their additional expertise and training.

The clinical nurse leader is an evolving role that has been developed over the past 10 years by the American Association of Colleges of Nurs-ing in conjuction with the larger education and practice communities. This role emerged as a response to the nursing shortage and the crisis in the health care system. There is a critical need to develop nurse leaders and to impact improvements in health outcomes. The focus of the role is described in the *White Paper on the Education and Role of the Clinical Nurse Leader* (AACN, 2007). "The CNL is a provider and a manager of care at the point of care to individuals and cohorts. The CNL designs, implements, and evaluates client care by coordinating, delegating and supervising the care provided by the health care team." The curriculum and core competencies of CNL education differ from APRN compe-tencies. As a result, APRN legislation does not apply to the CNL role. Graduates of CNL programs are licensed as registered nurses and are professionally certified as a CNL.

Within the traditional master's degree APRN preparation, there has been a trend in dual program enrollment or minors. Students may seek a specialty minor with an alternate clinical focus, such as pursuing a minor in acute care while enrolled in a primary care NP program. Students may not understand the extensive clinical requirements that must be completed in order to practice with a new population. These clinical requirements cannot be combined with their primary focus population and may require an additional 500 hours of training. While pursuing a minor in a different population may add a depth of personal knowledge, it does not lead to a change in the scope of practice. Students enrolled in dual programs (such as pediatrics and psychiatric/mental health) will need approximately 500 clinical hours in each area in order to be licensed/certified.

The current trends in nursing education and the evolution of the DNP and CNL reflect an exciting period of growth for nursing. Professional certification has been developed to recognize the CNL; however, as stated above, the CNL is not an APRN and, therefore, state legislation does not recognize these graduates as APRNs. The DNP is a graduate degree, just like the MSN or MS, and does not prepare an individual for one specific role. DNP programs may prepare individuals for entry into APRN practice. Therefore, an individual seeking recognition to practice as an APRN would also need to have national certification in that particular APRN role in order to be recognized to practice. In the future, licensing and credentialing may change to reflect the educational preparation of the APRN DNP.

ISSUES IN CREDENTIALING

Issues in Licensing

Licensure as a nurse and in some states as an advanced practice nurse assures that the individual who is granted the authority to practice nursing has demonstrated the cognitive, affective, and psychomotor competencies necessary for their role. Core licensure requirements for initial entry into the nursing profession are those minimum requirements that are essential to promote public protection. The majority of states and territories recognize the roles for advanced practice nursing by documenting the advanced graduate education and successful passing of a certification exam (also entry-level competence, or minimum requirement exam). Twenty-seven states recognize advanced practice with an additional license (National Council of State Boards of Nursing, 2007); other states and territories use certification, with only a few using registration or designation/recognition as an approach to regulation.

The future goal for nursing is to have uniform licensure requirements, which would be less confusing for patients, nurses, other health team members, and third-party payers. In addition, we hope that all states and territories will recognize advanced practice registered nurses with a second license (the highest form of regulation). With uniform core licensure requirements and advanced licensure requirements, the nurse is assured easier mobility across states and territories, while states maintain their licensure standards to protect the public. Health care consumers throughout the county are assured more access to nursing services and are assured that the nurse provider is qualified according to consistent standards.

It was not until the 1970s that licensure for registered nurses (RNs) and licensed practical nurses (LPNs) became mandatory in all U.S. jurisdictions (Weisenbeck & Calico, 1991). In 1996, advanced practice registered nurses were regulated by some method (licensure, certification, registration, or designation/recognition) in 49 of the 50 states (NCSBN, 2002). Because the purpose of licensure/regulation is the protection of the public, and the power to regulate professions (occupations) is based upon police power of the state to enact reasonable laws necessary to protect citizens, legislatures realized that expertise in the area being regulated was needed to develop more specific standards. Thus the concept of state boards/administrative agencies was born, and members of the regulated profession were used to provide the expertise needed to develop detailed requirements for the profession/occupation. Nurses must remember that one of the effects of physicians becoming the first health group licensed by the state is that there is the continuation of a legislative schema that grants physicians an exclusive and all-encompassing scope of practice for all things medical or health-related (Safriet, 1993). This creates an issue for advanced practice nursing legislation.

One can see, therefore, that when nurses perform acts that were traditionally part of medicine but are now considered nursing, there are controversies regarding licensure despite one's level of graduate education. Yet in the 21st century, some parents perform acts that were traditionally part of medicine and are now just parenting, like temperature taking to diagnose a fever or using an ear speculum to see if one's child has pain from an ear infection or foreign body in the ear canal.

Licensure and Graduate Education

So how will graduate education influence the license one would need to practice as an advanced practice registered nurse? It is important to remember the difference between academic degrees, programs of study leading to a particular nursing role, and advanced practice registered nurse roles that need to be recognized by state regulation in order to better protect the public and to increase consumer's access to competent health care services.

The DNP is an academic, professional nursing degree and can prepare both APRNs (certified nurse practitioners [CNPs], certified nurse midwives [CNMs], certified registered nurse anesthetists [CRNAs] or clinical nurse specialists [CNSs] and non-APRN graduates (administrators, public health nurses, informaticists, etc.). APRNs with a DNP degree, just as APRNs with master's degrees were required in the past, need state recognition, often a second license or certification, to practice in their expanded roles. Non-APRNs with a DNP are graduates with a professional doctorate that do not need additional state licensure or recognition beyond their RN license to practice with consumers, because they are practicing within the scope of practice of an RN and use their additional skill and knowledge in a different arena from APRNs.

The CNL is a new role in nursing practice that also does not require additional state recognition, for the scope of practice that is implemented as a CNL is within the traditional scope of practice of an RN. Once again the additional skill and knowledge obtained as a CNL, while studying for a master's degree in nursing, includes a different arena of competencies than the APRNs (CNP, CNM, CRNA, CNS) currently recognized in the United States.

APRNs currently recognized by states who have the professional doctorate (DNP) or the research doctorate (PhD, Doctorate of Nursing Science [DNSc], etc.) received their additional state license or recognition because of the scope of practice of the APRN role they were educated in, and by maintaining the needed second license or certification through meeting the state's requirements—most often national certification in the APRN role.

Movement from one state to another in one of the four APRN roles is at the discretion of the state. An APRN when moving must meet the current APRN criteria for practice in that state. An APRN who wants to move states would have to gain the additional education required by the state, before a license or certification is issued by that state—regardless if they have been practicing 20 years and have maintained national certification in the APRN role they wish to practice in the new state. The new APRN Regulatory Model recommends that individuals currently recognized to practice would be grandfathered in if moving to a new state as long as the criteria for recognition at the time of one's graduation met the new state's criteria at that time.

Grandfathering

Grandfathering is the term used by states to recognize current APRN providers in a state when state laws and regulation change. For example: prior to 2003, some CNPs were educated without a graduate degree, Master of Science in Nursing (MSN), but state law grandfathered them into continuing practice in the current state of employment. If that same person tried to move states, the new state would not necessarily recognize them as an APRN without a graduate degree. Twenty-four states require an MSN now (Christian, Denver, & O'Neil, 2007; Robitaille, 2008).

NCSBN has defined grandfathering as: "When states adopt new eligibility requirements for APRNs, currently practicing APRNs are permitted to continue to practice within the states in the APRN category through provisions recognized in most states. However, as stated earlier, the new APRN Regulatory Model recommends that individuals currently recognized to practice may be grandfathered in if moving to a new state as long as the criteria for recognition at the time of one's graduation met the new state's criteria at that time.

Scope of Practice

Licensed health care professionals' scope of practice is defined in each state's laws in the form of a practice act. The 1995 Pew Health Professions Commission report defined scope of practice as the "Definition of the rules, the regulations and boundaries within which a fully qualified practitioner with substantial and appropriate training, knowledge and experience may practice in a field of medicine or surgery, or other specifically defined field (i.e. nursing). Such practice is also governed by requirements for continuing education and professional accountability"

(Finocchio, Dower, McMahon, Gragnola, & the Task Force on Health Care Workforce Regulation, 1995; Sheets, 1996).

For example, CNPs prepared in continuing education programs in the late 1960s through 2002 were grandfathered into practice in the state they were currently recognized by a second license or some other recognition, such as a certificate in addition to their RN license. It took over 30 years to have all states mandate graduate education at the master's level for CNPs. The question arises: Will states in the next 30 years or less require a doctoral degree rather than the graduate master's degree? What usually happens is there is a coming together of all state boards, professional societies, educators, accreditors, and certifiers, and they propose a future date. Currently there is no uniform agreement on the year 2015 proposed by AACN for education programs to evolve to the DNP level preparing new APRNs (AACN, 2004; National Research Council of the National Academies, 2005). AACN gave us 10 years to change; it is more realistic to believe it will take 20 years, but hopefully not 30 or more, to bring about this recommendation.

We have already seen that the recommended scope of practice is expanded for the doctoral programs that prepare any of the four APRNs. (See NONPF and AACN's different views on scope of practice [AACN, 2004; NONPF, 2006]). Given the past history on changing scope of practice, it could be expected that by 2025, all new APRNs would be educated at the doctoral level, whether in the professional doctorate or research doctorate—they would meet the criterion on graduation from an academic program to receive an academic degree (DNP, PhD) and have met all the criterion to be prepared in an APRN role that they chose as part of their program of study. Thus they could sit for a national certification exam in a particular role.

Additional questions that remain for the state regulators, accreditors, certifiers, and educators are: How will each of these groups recognize the scope of practice of the APRN with a doctoral degree? Will states change state laws and rules and regulations to require doctoral rather than master's education for APRNs? We know educational institutions will always use the professional guidelines like the DNP competencies (AACN, 2004; NONPF, 2006) when developing new academic programs of study. And it can be expected that both CCNE and NLNAC will use the competencies outlined for APRN doctoral education to accredit existing and new practice doctorate programs of study. The PhD research degree in nursing has never been accredited by CCNE or NLNAC since it was not focused on preparing DNPs.

Based on graduation from a doctoral program that has prepared a student in one of the four APRN roles (whether DNP or PhD), students would be eligible to submit their credentials to an organization that offers national certification in a particular APRN role and population, such as pediatric nurse practitioners (PNCB, ANCC). The certification organization would review their applications and approve them to sit for the national exam. The question arises as to whether the graduate of a doctoral program will take the same exam for an APRN role and population as a graduate from a master's program. It is expected that the required additional competences for the doctorate will also be tested. Whether the competencies are integrated into a new exam or through an additional module of new expanded scope of practice questions based on the additional doctoral competencies has not been decided.

One question that continues to persist focuses on the verbal use of the title *Doctor* by doctorally prepared nurses. Scrutiny of professional state law is required to answer this query. The number of states prohibiting the use of *Doctor* varies from one (Illinois) to nine (Klein, 2007), depending on the written source. The use of this title does not negate the nursing profession. Nurses may be proud of their role but choose to use *Doctor* as recognition of their advanced education. A doctorally prepared nurse may introduce herself as "I am Doctor Mary Smith, a pediatric nurse practitioner because I have a doctoral degree—I am not a medical doctor such as a pediatrician. But don't be surprised when you hear people call me Dr. Mary."

ISSUES IN CERTIFICATION

Certifying Bodies

A number of professional organizations provide certification to advanced practice registered nurses (see Table 10.1). To be eligible to sit for these exams, one needs to be an RN and complete a graduate-level accredited education program. The exam chosen must correspond to the type of program completed and must test beginning competencies for entry-level practitioners. Additionally, a wide diversity of certification exams exist for master's-prepared nurses in value-added specialty areas (see Table 10.2). Many of these exams are designed to test expert level competencies.

Table 10.1

ORGANIZATIONS CERTIFYING APRN ROLES

PROFESSIONAL ORGANIZATION	ACRONYM	CERTIFYING ORGANIZATION	ACRONYM	TYPE OF APRN
American Association of Critical Care Nurses	AACN	American Association of Critical Care Nurses Certification Corporation	AACNCC	CNP CNS
American Nurses Association	ANA	American Nurses Credentialing Center	ANCC	CNP CNS
American Association of Nurse Anesthetists	AANA	Council on Certification of Nurse Anesthetists	CCNA	CRNA
American College of Nurse Midwives	ACNM	American Midwifery Certification Board	AMCB	CNM
American Academy of Nurse Practitioners	AANP	American Academy of Nurse Practitioners Certification Program	AANPCP	CNP
Association for Woman's Health, Obstetric and Neonatal Nurses	AWHONN	National Certification Corporation for Obstetric, Gynecologic, & Neonatal Nursing Specialties	NCC	CNP
National Association of Pediatric Nurse Practitioners	NAPNAP	Pediatric Nursing Certification Board (formerly NCBPNP/N)	PNCB	CNP

Table 10.2

EXAMPLES OF VALUE-ADDED CERTIFICATION

PROFESSIONAL ORGANIZATION	ACRONYM	CERTIFYING ORGANIZATION	ACRONYM	VALUE ADDED CERTIFICATION
Oncology Nursing Society	ONS	Oncology Nurse Certification Corporation	ONCC	Oncology
National Association of Orthopedic Nurses	NAON	Orthopedic Nurse Certification Board	ONCB	Orthopedics
American Nurses Association	ANA	American Nurses Credentialing Center	ANCC	Diabetes/Pain Management, for example
American Nephrology Nurses Association	ANNA	Nephrology Nursing Certification Commission	NNCC	Nephrology

Uses of Certification

National certification is used for a variety of different types of credentialing. A preponderance of state boards have adopted professional certification rather than an academic degree to recognize advanced nursing practice. Although certification through professional organizations is voluntary, some states require passing a voluntary exam and submitting the results to be included in the materials necessary to receive a form of additional recognition such as a certificate or license. National certification is one part of the licensing requirement for nurses in an APRN role. Standardized national certification exams exist for each of the four direct care provider APRN roles: CNP, CNM, CRNA, and CNS.

CNS licensure/certification is especially problematic, because the examinations given by certifiers are often administered to smaller numbers and therefore are not psychometrically sound and legally defensible. Additionally, not every CNS specialty has an examination, although the majority of states now require APRNs to be nationally certified. The

National Association of Clinical Nurse Specialists argue in their 2003 position paper that this policy is fine for CNPs, CNMs, and CRNAs, roles with a medical domain in their practice, but they feel that the CNS role falls under the purview of the RN license and that mandatory certification or second licensure is not necessary. Since many specialties do not have examinations, it has been proposed that alternate mechanisms for demonstrating competency, such as portfolios, peer review, or continuing education be utilized. Even though many CNSs feel that developing a single CNS exam is an unacceptable solution, as of this writing ANCC and the National Association of Clinical Nurse Specialists (NACNS) are developing a core CNS exam for the role and for each population foci. This will cover "critical elements of CNS practice" for CNSs practicing in specialty areas that have no certification exam available.

All APRNs who have been certified in a role (CNP, CNM, CRNA, CNS) and population area (pediatrics, neonatal, adult/gerontology, psych mental health, women's health/gender related, or Family/individual across the life span) may take value-added specialty certification exams to add to their resume and achieve additional professional recognition and competence. For example, someone licensed and certified as an adult nurse practitioner could chose to obtain additional certification in occupational health or oncology.

All nurses with graduate degrees are not necessarily APRNs. Certification is also available for master's or doctorally prepared nurses who do not provide direct patient care. Voluntary certification in an area such as diabetes could be available to nurses with a graduate degree in leadership as a measure of special expertise to be used in patient education.

As mentioned earlier, the CNL role and practice model is not an APRN role; therefore, graduates of these programs are not eligible for APRN licensure. Beginning in 2007, AACN administered a certification examination for nurses educated as CNLs. Only those individuals who successfully pass the CNL certification examination and maintain certification are eligible to use the title CNL.

Upon careful review of the certifying organizations that have certification exams available for APRNs, none currently has a position statement on the DNP, however, all of the APRN certification bodies have stated they do allow DNP graduates to sit for certification if the program prepares the graduate for entry into APRN practice. But some of the affiliated professional associations (such as The American Academy of Nurse Practitioners [AANP] and the National Association of Clinical Nurse Specialists [NACNS]) do have statements or at least discussion points regarding the DNP. AACN urges the certifying organizations to incorporate the DNP essentials into the APRN certification mechanisms. The eligibility criteria to apply for APRN certification includes an RN license and a master's, post-master's, or doctoral degree from an accredited APRN role and population program. Therefore, nurse graduates from an approved DNP program with content that meets national criteria for education in an APRN role (CNS, CNP, CRNA, and CNM) will be eligible for licensure/certification.

Future Issues in Certification

- Should the certifying exam for DNP graduates be the same as the one offered to master's graduates of APRN role programs?
- Will all of the national certification exams be able to meet the high-stakes criteria to be psychometrically sound and legally defensible?
- Will the APRN exam for doctoral graduates be offered as an additional module to the MSN exam or as an entirely new APRN doctoral exam?

Issues in Employer/Institutional Credentialing

Advanced practice registered nurses are credentialed through state licensure/regulation and professional certifying organizations that recognize competency. However, in order to practice in a health care institution or affiliate, a third layer of credentialing must be completed. Employer institutional credentialing is required of all licensed APRNs in order to gain the privilege to practice in that facility. Institutions mandate credentialing of practitioners in order to protect the public and ensure safety and quality of care. Such institutions include hospitals, outpatient health centers, long-term care facilities, and schools and universities. Managed care agencies and insurance companies also require credentialing of all practitioners prior to inclusion on a participating provider panel or list.

Institutions are required to meet credentialing standards set by national accrediting organizations such as The Joint Commission (TJC). There are several national organizations that set standards for credentialing providers, including government agencies such as the Health Resources and Services Administration (HRSA), the Centers for Medicare and Medicaid Services (CMS), and the Bureau of Primary Health Care (BPHC). In addition, private agencies that offer credentialing standards and services include the National Committee for Quality Assurance (NCQA), the Accreditation Association for Ambulatory Health Care (AAAHC), and the Utilization Review Accreditation Commission (URAC).

TJC is a well-respected source of specific standards for credentialing health care providers. In order for institutions to gain accreditation with TJC these standards must be met. TJC defines credentialing as the process of obtaining, verifying, and assessing the qualifications of a health care practitioner to provide patient or resident care services in or for a health care organization (TJC, 2004). These qualifications include documented evidence of licensure, education, training, and experience. An organization must credential all licensed independent practitioners on an ongoing basis. TJC provides comprehensive guidelines for credentialing through an evidence-based process that must be used by employer institutions.

Institutional credentialing is a complex process for each practitioner. Upon initial employment the institution must verify information about work history, experience, education, physical health, mental health, criminal and drug history, history with the licensing board, previous malpractice suits and settlements, malpractice insurance, and current employment by other institutions. If any of these areas are found to be inadequate, the employer will not grant practice privileges to the practitioner.

Part of the institutional credentialing requirement includes an ongoing professional practice evaluation. Organizations are obligated to maintain current information on each provider, including APRN licensure, national certification data, and updated continuing education information. Periodically the credentialing process must be repeated. In addition, a focused practice evaluation is required, which examines the quality of care provided by the practitioner. This may be achieved through quality improvement measures such as chart review or outcomes data measurement.

HRSA is a federal agency of the U.S. Department of Health and Human Services. The goal of this organization is to improve access to health care for individuals who are uninsured, isolated, or medically vulnerable. The HSRA collaborates with the Bureau of Primary Health Care (BPHC) and states that a health center credentialing process should meet the standards of a national accrediting organization such as TJC.

The National Practitioner Data Bank (NPDB) and the Healthcare Integrity and Protection Data Bank (HIPDB) are federally managed data banks, which can be used by employer institutions during the process of credentialing. The Health Care Quality Improvement Act of 1986 led to the development of the NPDB. It provides information that may be used to identify practitioners who engage in unprofessional behavior, are incompetent, or are involved in a malpractice suit. The HIPDB was created as part of the Health Insurance Portability and Accountability Act of 1996. The focus of this data bank is to provide important information about the past actions of practitioners and involvement in fraud and abuse in health care delivery.

Institutions must credential all licensed practitioners, including RNs and APRNs. Since the process is dependent on licensure, only those APRNs with a separate license or certificate are credentialed separately from RNs. These include CNSs, CNPs, CRNAs, and CNMs. The DNP degree and the CNL role are not recognized through separate licensure/certification by the state board of nursing. Therefore they are not credentialed separately. Such individuals would be credentialed as an RN unless they met the qualifications of an APRN with separate licensure/certification.

Managed care agencies and insurance companies credential practitioners in order to enroll them as providers in their health plans. This allows practitioners to directly or indirectly receive reimbursement for health care services rendered. Managed care agencies and insurance companies grant privileges to providers, including APRNs who are licensed/certified to provide reimbursable clinical services. Individuals holding a DNP degree would be enrolled as providers if they met the qualifications of an APRN and hold an APRN license.

IMPACT OF CREDENTIALING ON CLINICAL PRACTICE

The next few years will be an exciting time and bring much change for all of us. Some very exciting news includes the completion of a new paper on the legislative, accreditation, certification, and educational (LACE) process to be used for future credentialing of all APRNs. This paper is the result of 4 years of work of the APRN Consensus Work Group and the National Council of State Boards of Nursing APRN Committee. In addition, as of March 2008 the NCSBN APRN Committee introduced the language of the Model Act rules and regulations for all APRNs based on the language of this new joint dialogue paper. Progressive states where APRNs are autonomous, educational institutions, accrediting organizations, and certifying organizations have fostered delivery models of practice that suggest that the public is better served with high-quality and efficient care that is readily accessible through APRNs. We currently have a maldistribution of health care providers, although it is understandable why APRNs would prefer to practice in progressive states. Now is the time from all reports (Institute of Medicine [IOM], Pew NCSBN) for more interprofessional collaboration while maintaining autonomy for each profession. With it, consumers and providers alike will benefit, and legislators will be relieved from wrestling with questions regarding the health of the public that they are not necessarily prepared to debate.

Because the historical interest of boards of medicine (protecting physicians' interests) are inherently in conflict with the interests of boards of nursing (protecting nursing interests), collaboration will be difficult, but with both professions caring about what is best for the public without compromising quality and safety, success is to be expected over time (California HealthCare Foundation, 2008).

REFERENCES

American Association of Colleges of Nursing. (2004). *AACN position statement on the practice doctorate in nursing.* Washington, DC: Author.

American Association of Colleges of Nursing. *Essentials of doctoral education for advanced nursing practice.* Retrieved July 13, 2008 from American Association of Colleges of Nursing website: http://www.aacn.nche.edu/DNP/index.htm

American Association of Colleges of Nursing. (2007). *AACN white paper on CNL education and role of clinical nurse leader.* Retrieved January 16, 2008, from aacn.nche. edu/Publications/whitepaers/ClinicalNurseLeader07.pdf

American Nurses' Association. (1955). ANA board approves a definition of nursing practice. *American Nurses' Association, 55,* 1474.

American Nurses' Association. (1979). Credentialing in nursing. A new approach: Report of the committee for the study of credentialing in nursing. *American Journal of Nursing, 79,* 674–683.

Bullough, B. (1982). State certification of nursing specialties: A new trend in nursing practice law. *Pediatric Nursing, 8,* 121–124.

California HealthCare Foundation. (2008). *Scope of practice laws in healthcare: Rethinking the role of nurse practitioners.* Oakland, CA: Author.

Christian, S., Denver, C., & O'Neil, E. (2007). *Overview of nurse practitioner scopes of practice in the United States—Discussion.* USCF Centers for the Health professions. Retrieved February 7, 2008, from http://futurehealth.ucsf.edu

Dorroh, M. W., & Kelley, M. A. (2005). The certified nurse-midwife. In A. B. Hamric, J. A. Spross, & C. M. Hanson (Eds.), *Advanced practice nursing: An integrative approach* (pp. 551–581). St. Louis, MO: Elsevier Saunders.

Finocchio, L. J., Dower, C. M., McMahon, T., Gragnola, C. M., & the Task Force on Health Care Workforce Regulation. (1995). *Reforming health care workforce regulation: Policy considerations for the 21st Century.* San Francisco: Pew Health Professions Commission.

Hanson, C. M. (2005). Understanding regulatory, legal and credentialing requirements. In A. B. Hamric, J. A. Spross, & C. M. Hanson (Eds.), *Advanced practice nursing: An integrative approach* (pp. 781–808). St. Louis, MO: Elsevier Saunders.

The Joint Commission. (2004). *The medical staff handbook: A guide to Joint Commission standards* (2nd ed.). Oakbrook Terrace, IL: Joint Commission Resources.

The Joint Commission. (2008). *A journey through the history of the Joint Commissions.* Retrieved January 28, 2008, from www.jointcommision.org/AboutUs/joint_commission_history.htm

Jones, D. C. (2002). Reimbursement, privileging and credentialing for pediatric nurse practitioners. *Medscape.* Retrieved January 30, 2008, from www.medscape.com/view article/433372

Klein, T. (2007). Are nurses with a Doctor of Nursing Practice degree called "Doctor"? *Medscape.* Retrieved February 1, 2008, from www.medscape.com/viewarticle/563176

McAtee, P. A., & Silver, H. K. (1974). Nurse practitioners for children—Past and future. *Pediatrics, 54,* 578–582.

McLeod, R. (1995). Nurse practitioners: Building on our past to meet future challenges. *Advanced Practice Nursing Quarterly, 1,* 15–20.

McGivern, D. O., Sullivan-Marx, E. M., & Mezey, M. D. (2003). Advanced practice nursing: Preparation and clinical practice. In M. D. Mezey, D. O. McGivern, & E. M. Sullivan-Marx (Eds.), *Nurse practitioners: Evolution of advanced practice* (4th ed., pp. 3–36). New York: Springer Publishing.

Millonig, V. L. (1986). Considering pediatric nurse practitioner certification. *Pediatric Nursing, 12,* 268–290.

National Association of Clinical Nurse Specialists. (2003). NACNS position paper: Regulatory credentialing of clinical nurse specialists. *Clinical Nurse Specialist, 17,* 163–169.

National Council of State Boards of Nursing. (1993). *Position paper on the regulation of advanced nursing practice.* Retrieved January 15, 2008, from https://www.ncsbn.org/1993_Position_Paper_on_the_Regulation_of_Advanced_Nursing_Practice.pdf

National Council of State Boards of Nursing. (2002). *Regulation of advanced practice nursing. NCSBN position paper.* Retrieved February 2, 2008, from www.ncsbn.org/APRN_Position_Paper2002.pdf

National Council of State Boards of Nursing. (2007). *Changes in healthcare professions scope of practice: Legislative considerations.* Retrieved January 3, 2008, from http://www.ncsbn.org/scopeofpractice

National Organization of Nurse Practitioner Faculties. (2006). *Practice doctorate nurse practitioner entry level competences.* Retrieved February 2, 2008, from http://www.nonpf.com/NONPF2005/PracticeDoctorateResourceCenter/PDResourceCenter.htm

National Research Council of the National Academies. (2005). *Advancing the nation's health needs: NIH research training programs.* Washington, DC: National Academies Press.

National Task Force on Quality Nurse Practitioner Education. (2008). *Criteria for evaluation of nurse practitioner programs.* Retrieved July 13, 2008 from the National

Organization of Nurse Practitioner Faculties web site: http://www.nonpf.org/NONPF2005/NTFCriteriaWebVersion0208.pdf

Porcher, F. K. (2003). Licensure, certification and credentialing. In M. D. Mezey, D. O. McGivern, & E. M. Sullivan-Marx (Eds.), *Nurse practitioners: Evolution of advanced practice* (4th ed., pp. 415–429). New York: Springer Publishing.

Robitaille, S. (2008). *Scope of practice laws in health care: Rethinking the role of nurse practitioners.* Issue Brief from California Healthcare Foundation, Oakland, CA. Retrieved January 31, 2008, from http://www.chcf.org/topics/view.cfm?itemid=133568

Safriet, B. J. (1993). *One strong voice.* Keynote address presented at the National Nurse Practitioner Leadership Summit, February 1993, Washington, DC.

Safriet, B. J. (2002). Closing the gap between can and may in health-care providers' scope of practice: A primer for policy makers. *Yale Journal on Regulation, 19,* 301–334.

Sheets, V. (1996). *Protection or profession self-preservation? The purpose of regulation.* Chicago: National Council of State Boards of Nursing.

Weisenbeck, S., & Calico, P. A. (1991). Licensure and related issues in nursing. In G. Deloughere (Ed.), *Issues and trends in nursing* (pp. 243–277). St. Louis, MO: Mosby Company.

11

Voices From the Field: The Doctor of Nursing Practice Degree

MARY T. QUINN GRIFFIN, HELEN A. GORDON, AND COLLEEN A. MAYKUT

The Doctor of Nursing Practice (DNP) is a relatively new practice-focused degree in nursing. The American Association of Colleges of Nursing (AACN) has published a position statement identifying the DNP as the degree for practice-focused doctoral education in nursing. At Case Western Reserve University (Case) this is offered at a number of different entry points either as direct entry or at the post-master's level. In this chapter the two students sharing their experiences are in the post-master's program. In this program there are two tracks, the clinical leadership track and the educational leadership track. The clinical leadership track prepares doctoral students for clinical positions as administrators and direct care providers, while the educational leadership track focuses on preparation for educators in either academic or clinical positions. Students in both these tracks receive core education in health policy and in research. Additionally, the education track provides courses in curriculum and instruction, testing and evaluation, and a teaching practicum. The leadership track has courses in management, advanced practice, information management, and organizational behavior. Graduates with a DNP degree are the most highly qualified practitioners in nursing. These graduates use their education and expertise to lead the profession in practice situations where patients have increasing levels of complexity and have a major role in managing and responding to the intricacies of the health care industry itself.

In this chapter early adopters of this program share their experiences and future plans. They each have a unique perspective even though they chose the education track in the program. The first student is a faculty member at Duke University and is at the beginning of her course work. Information about their experiences with the DNP curriculum and their future plans will help us to build and revise programs to meet the growing needs of the DNP graduates. The second student is an international student from Canada who is certainly at the forefront of Canadian nursing, as she will be one of the first DNP-prepared nurses in Canada. These voices provide valuable insights as to the education practice arenas these students will embrace and shape when they graduate from the DNP program.

These students wished to make a difference to nursing education in particular, but also to practice. They identified their need and desire for further education to broaden their teaching knowledge and skills while acquiring further knowledge in areas related to their practice. One of the strengths of this chapter is that the students share their reasons for pursuing the DNP degree and their future plans. They relate how the DNP provided the best educational fit for them, as they did not have any desire to pursue a research-focused doctorate. Furthermore, the DNP program provided opportunities to network with nursing leaders as well as with peers within the program, as it has students with many different levels of experience from a wide variety of practice and academic settings throughout the United States. One tremendous advantage identified by these students was that all of the courses are offered in the intensive format. This means the content for each course is taught during one 6-day period with the course assignments submitted throughout the semester. Some of the courses have an online portion. Lessons learned for future DNP programs are that this is a very successful format for students at this level, as it is easier for these students to schedule their course work while working in their regular employment. In addition it provides the face-to-face-contact and interaction lacking in online-only courses, and, most importantly, it facilitates networking. Barriers for the students at this level are the cost of these programs, particularly as these students have invested heavily in their education throughout their careers, and they are at a stage in their personal lives that has costs incurred for family. The DNP program offers practitioners a doctoral education that is practice-focused and is specifically designed to meet their career trajectory. This program has proven itself to be innovative and practical and is the program of choice for clinical nurse leaders in education and practice.

ONE PROFESSION, MANY CAREERS: HELEN A. GORDON

Educational Program Perspectives

Background of My Career Trajectory

I have been a nurse for 33 years. Following my graduation in 1974 I realized my practice "love" was maternity. In 1976, my goal was to be a nurse-midwife, and I hoped along the way to gain some experience with different cultures, as I had been raised in an extremely homogeneous, small rural community and had no experience with different cultures. At the time of my admission to graduate school at Utah, Dr. Madeline Lenninger was the dean of nursing. After completing her introductory course in nursing theory and being assigned to a clinical practicum on a Navaho Indian reservation in Shiprock, New Mexico for 12 weeks, I declared that my goals had been met.

Over the course of the next 30 years I did many things with my degrees in nursing and midwifery. I practiced nurse-midwifery for 4 years. Leaving clinical practice for a more balanced lifestyle for my family, I was a head nurse, the director of two obstetrical units. As a director I established the first labor, delivery, recovery, post-partum (LDRP) unit in the United States at St. Mary's Hospital (now Riverside Medical Center) in Minneapolis, Minnesota. I was then recruited to design and implement the first tertiary LDRP in Raleigh, North Carolina at WakeMed Health and Hospitals. These combined experiences positioned me strongly for a job with a women's health consulting firm in Salt Lake City. From 1989 to 1992, I was the senior consultant, having worked with an estimated 30 hospitals in some capacity over 4 years as a coach and a consultant in the design and implementation of contemporary, competitive, market-driven, family-centered maternity units.

Changes in my family structure, specifically the addition of a new baby in 1992–1993, challenged me to stay closer to home. For 5 years I was the obstetrical program specialist for the North Carolina Office of Rural Health. I was assigned to grow nurse-midwifery practices and expand existing opportunities for nurse-midwives in North Carolina. In

1998, this position ended and I joined the staff of the American College of Nurse-Midwives (ACNM). At a satellite office in North Carolina I managed American College of Nurse-Midwives' (ACNM) first Providers Partnership Grant funding through the Maternal Child Health (MCH) Bureau. I directly coached and oversaw the establishment of partnerships between state Certified Nurse Midwifes (CNM) and Title 10 directors in 10 states. This position ended in 2000 and I pursued my own independent consulting for the next 3 years, combining this with two shifts a week at a medical center as a staff nurse in labor-delivery. All this is background to say that by the time I had reached 2006 I had 30 years of varied and eclectic experience in nursing. This experience I termed "one profession with many careers."

Transition to Academia

In early 2005, I was invited to be the contract faculty for the summer for the Duke School of Nursing's maternity course in their accelerated bachelor of nursing program. From the first moment I stepped into that classroom I was "in love" with teaching these second degree students. They were bright, inquisitive, demanding, and focused. Drawing on my years as a childbirth educator and teaching nursing staff member, it tapped every ounce of creativity I had in me to make theoretical concepts in the classroom relevant to their clinical experience. At that time this program was still in embryonic stages of development, so I had few visual aids or films to use. I consistently improvised from readily accessible aids that I developed to address the educational needs of students. It seemed the more homemade teaching tools I could dream up the better the students loved it. They told me that my teaching strategies helped them bridge the classroom to the clinical. For me the opportunity fueled my creativity like nothing I had ever experienced in my work life. I became hooked on the notion that I was a midwife "birthing" new nurses to the profession. I said it was a calling like none other I had experienced.

After that summer I inquired regarding the still vacant faculty position, only to be told again that the search committee was holding out for a PhD candidate. I was disappointed, but what could I do? I was not doctorally prepared. Then in December of 2005 two critical incidents occurred. The outgoing students, the ones I had taught that first summer, created and voted me the first ever "faculty of the year" in the program. The second event was that the search committee had failed to produce an acceptable PhD candidate for the permanent position.

Now again, 6 months away from the summer maternity course, I was invited and this time *encouraged* to apply for the faculty position. The combination of the national shortage of faculty and my positive summer outcomes gave me the entrance ticket into this prestigious institution.

I joined the faculty; however, I was clear during my final negotiation meeting that I had no intention at my age of pursuing doctoral education. Also I just had too much financial responsibility as my children were in college and I really had no interest in going back to school or conducting nursing research. I felt my newly found niche was teaching. The dean agreed with my plan and said that with the shortage of available faculty and my extensive background in maternity nursing, my skills were more than adequate, and I would more than likely be quite comfortable finishing out my nursing career as a master's-level faculty member at Duke.

Here Comes the DNP

Happy, excited, and naive, I embarked on the next phase of my professional trajectory. All seemed quite blissful till the end of the summer of 2006 when three critical events occurred. These coalesced to make me decide to return to school. First, my course evaluations from the students were not as stellar as the previous year, with some students harshly criticizing both my style and my methods. While my course evaluations were still acceptable, I felt I had lost my edge from the previous year. On reflection, I had not been able to assess and diagnose the learning style difference in this current group of students, but additionally I felt I had nothing in my "tool kit" of teaching strategies that gave me a frame of reference for understanding what had gone wrong. My confidence was severely shaken.

Secondly, in late August the Accelerated Bachelor of Science in Nursing (ABSN) program moved into the newly constructed school of nursing. This move positioned all the school of nursing faculty under one roof. I noticed a marked change in the dynamics of interacting with the other faculty. My new inherited colleagues, most of whom were PhD nurse researchers, seemed to clearly be the "power brokers" in the building, the ones that both spoke and commanded the attention that goes with the faculty rank, tenure, and research dollars. While understandable, it was still somewhat curious to me.

The final tipping point in mid-fall was the announcement that our School of Nursing planned to start a Doctorate of Nursing Practice program. My interest was now moved beyond curious, it was *piqued*. After considerable research into all the AACN-listed DNP programs in the United States, I decided this might be a feasible path for me. I came to the conclusion that with the right program plan I could strengthen what I perceived as my teaching weaknesses, begin to build a base of evidence for what worked in teaching, and perhaps secure my faculty position. To me this meant that with a doctorate I would be able to continue to direct the creation and management of my own courses. I figured that with a jump start of a year, I might be in a position to be of value in the new DNP program if I were prepared at this.

So my plan to pursue a DNP degree began to take shape. I knew I needed a specific kind of DNP program to meet my personal needs. I had no intention of leaving my current position, and I knew I needed a program that had the flexibility to allow me to continue teaching full-time, but it could not be a program that was online. Most of all I knew that I wanted to be impacted by the minds of the professors and students at this level of thinking. From having attempted an on-line course in the past, I did not and still do not believe this can happen in a totally on-line environment. I searched for only that program that would meet my criteria.

Educational Preparation

In early 2007, guided by the steady support of my mentor and a number of senior faculty, I applied to Case Western Reserve University's program in the educational leadership track. Within 6 weeks I was accepted into the program. I could not have been more pleased. The courses were stimulating, informative, and more than anything have revealed those areas of my own knowledge blind spots. I did not know what I did not know about the scholarship of teaching nursing.

I started the DNP with the goal of transforming my teaching. I wished to learn the foundational evidence for teaching adults and learning as adults in this new technology age. I wanted more than anything to be able to bridge the complexities of patient care that students encounter in the acute hospital and community environments with the best of nursing theory and research. Finally, my goal was to develop myself as a master teacher and a consumer and interpreter of nursing research.

The unexpected outcome has been how much fun it has been to be a *mature* student. The joy that has come from mastering the logistics of traveling to Case three times a year, to delving into the contemporary readings and course work and the exposure to the incredible scholarship and mentoring that has come from being at a school like Case with leaders in the profession. The Case DNP program not only offers class sizes that are small, but the students who comprise this rich student body in the DNP come from all backgrounds and areas of the world. As a student I have the opportunity to interact one on one with professors and collaborate on projects and publications. I just never expected this kind of mentoring.

One of the largest surprises has been the reaction of my students. Not only have they been willing partners and positive evaluators as I tried out many new teaching methodologies, they tell me I have been a role model. As one of them said at the end of fall semester, "you have shown me that not only can I be anything I want to be in nursing, but your return to school at *your age* has taught me that learning never has to stop in the profession."

Summary and Future Directions

It has been a great journey. Only nursing would offer the incredible flexibility to have worn so many "hats" in the profession. To this now 56-year-old woman, soon to complete a doctorate in nursing, I would say it has been more than worth the effort. I expect I will finish out my career, hopefully in my seventies, feeling well prepared to hold my faculty rank. Hopefully I will have progressed in my work by moving up the clinical track and, more importantly, I will be confident that I am providing to my students the best I can give in the application of contemporary research and teaching. I will owe this to my doctorate preparation.

As one of my Duke colleagues, Dr. Judith Hays, said, and Dean May Wykle at Case echoed, "With the DNP you will have put the evidence to what was, at one time, just your hunches about teaching."

A CANADIAN DNP STUDENT SPEAKS: COLLEEN A. MAYKUT

Educational Program Perspectives

There are numerous reasons why I decided to pursue a Doctorate in Nursing Practice (DNP) degree. Not least among them is the fact that there is a growing shortage of doctorally prepared nurses (Canadian Nurses Association [CNA] & Canadian Association of Schools of

Nursing [CASN], 2004; McKenna, 2005; Meleis & Dracup, 2005; Pastor, Cimiotti, & Stone, 2004). Although doctoral programs in Canada are recently established when compared to the United States, there is a strong mandate to increase enrollment to ensure nurses are available for research, academia, and leadership roles (CASN, 2006; CNA & CASN, 2004; Thorne, 2006). Canada has a small population of doctorally prepared nurses; 0.4% of the registered nurse population is the projected target for the year 2014 (CASN, 2006). This shortage has an impact on the development of nursing knowledge and the future education of students (CASN, 2006; CNA & CASN, 2004; Meleis & Dracup, 2005). I could see this and wished to make a difference to Canadian nursing education particularly, and also to practice.

When going through the decision process I had many conversations with nurses about the pros and cons of the DNP degree. Concerns with the DNP emerged from a variety of areas. Those opposed to this degree suggested that there will be a decrease in enrollment of PhD students, that it deters focus from crucial nursing issues, that it confuses stakeholders (the public, other nurses, health care professionals), and that to date there is no consensus in the United States with respect to the necessity of the DNP-prepared graduate (Fulton & Lyon, 2005; Meleis & Dracup, 2005). These oppositions were disputed strongly by the defenders of the DNP.

One key influential advantage I recognized in comparing the DNP to the PhD is the potential ability to minimize the theory–practice gap, as it is a practice-based professional doctorate. The DNP program is unique in the way it offers innovative approaches to clinical or educational issues and prepare graduates for clinical or educational leadership roles (AACN, 2004; Bunkers, 2002; Loomis, Williard, & Cohen, 2005; O'Sullivan, Carter, Marion, Pohl, & Werner, 2005; Yam, 2005). I was excited to read that Boyer (1996) has broadened the original concept of the scholastic excellence concept to include teaching as scholarly excellence. This helped me to make the final decision to pursue the DNP, because I was interested in developing educational excellence as I was nursing faculty.

Other discussions focused on the DNP's lack of scientific inquiry, rigor, and scholastic preparation for a teaching position in academia (Meleis & Dracup, 2005). When I investigated the DNP at Case Western Reserve University I was pleased to find that the program was strong in scientific inquiry and rigor. The program offers two unique streams, depending on the student's career path; educational leadership and clinical leadership (Francis Payne Bolton School of Nursing [FPB], 2007–2008a). The Educational Leadership track focuses on curriculum development, evaluation, and teaching strategies, key aspects to assist academic faculty (FPB, 2007–2008a). This track seemed exactly what I needed to meet my personal goals as nursing faculty. All of the courses are offered in the intensive format, that is, the course content is taught in a 6-day period and the assignments are submitted throughout the semester. Some courses are supplemented with on-line components.

Weighing both sides of the DNP debate and scrutinizing educational institutions with respect to the previously decisive factors, a clear choice became apparent. The Frances Payne Bolton School of Nursing at Case surpassed the previous criteria from this student's perspective (FPB 2007–2008b; FPB Centers of Excellence, n.d.). The DNP program at Case, with a focus on educational leadership and curriculum development, was chosen for a number of personal and professional reasons. Professionally, the program has a solid reputation for research and has a long history of grooming influential nursing leaders. As a Canadian nurse this international program offered an additional perspective not available in Canada and an occasion to network with leaders of nursing and colleagues. Professional networks created occasions to discuss with other nursing clinicians/educators the areas for improvement in our chosen fields. Specifically, the educational leadership track produced the opportunity to develop mock curricula to influence upcoming nursing generations and engage in nursing research to ensure effective nursing education.

Transition to Professional Role

The DNP program at Case was able to assist in my enrichment as a student with prior experience as nursing faculty. Progressing through the program, prior experience was valued, and I was able to develop and grow in all areas of the educational leadership track, but particularly in the areas I identified as having the greatest needs. On a personal note, my transition from clinician to a professional academic role was not straightforward. There have been barriers as well as facilitators along the journey. As an advanced nurse practitioner (ANP) graduate, clinical expertise was obtained at the expense of minimal teaching competencies. However, my clinical expertise has benefited me in my nursing faculty role and in turn the nursing students during both theory and clinical courses. The lack of teaching focus during the ANP program imposed a barrier during the transition from clinician to the role of nursing faculty. Therefore, further education with a focus on teaching theory and skills was deemed to be not just beneficial but essential for my professional growth. However, barriers once again existed during the educational experience.

Personally, specific barriers of the DNP program included the physical distance, having to travel from western Canada to either San Diego or Cleveland (some of the Case courses were offered in San Diego). Another major barrier was the financial burden of the tuition (the cost of a private American university versus a Canadian government-subsidized institution), and the travel and accommodation costs. One distinct disadvantage was the prominent American–Canadian differences with respect to academia and the health care system. Specific examples include entrance requirements for nursing, and health care policies. However, exposure to different viewpoints from faculty and peer-students, as well as innovative teaching and learning strategies, strengthened the student's academia portfolio.

Facilitators of this educational journey included the stimulating culture within FPB at Case, which was supportive and conducive to learning, resulting in acquisition of practical knowledge to inform current practice. The design of the DNP program was very appealing, a distinctive and unusual scholastic model to fit individual needs. The intensive format allowed for minimal disruption between professional and personal life. There are also cohorts, where groups of approximately 10 students enrolled in the DNP program, at the same time, take many of the courses in their home area with the FPB faculty traveling to them. These cohorts created two benefits: financial costs were decreased with faculty bringing courses to the students, and increased professional and personal collaboration as well as support between students. Overall, the DNP program at Case offered a superior reputation for scholastic achievement, supportive and enthusiastic nursing faculty, a successful marriage between clinical expertise and curriculum knowledge, and a flexible schedule to ensure student satisfaction.

Educational Preparation

Nursing education must incorporate evidence-based practice, up-to-date technology, and innovative strategies to ensure currency and credibility (CNA, 2002; Davis, 2006). These concepts were reinforced through the courses offered at FPB. The ability to incorporate diverse knowledge into my practice in education is a significant asset when facilitating student learning. One challenge for me as nursing faculty member is to keep up to date with the ever-evolving technical world; as nursing faculty I must be proactive instead of reactive to new forms of knowledge delivery (Chandra & Paul, 2004; Doutrich, Hoeksel, Wykoff, & Thiele, 2005; Johnson, 2001). Although historically there has been an interest in new delivery options—discussion rooms, distance learning, Web-based learning (Johnson, 2001; Moore et al., 2006; Polhamus, Farel, & Trester, 2000); comfort and competence levels in educators has been low (Polhamus, Farel & Trester, 2000). An increase in comfort may be a positive indicator for lifelong learning in both faculty and students with respect to technology (Moore et al., 2006; Polhamus, Farel, & Trester, 2000). I know that my comfort level with technology has increased as I enhanced my skills and explored new technologies during my course work. Information technology and information literacy skills have now become a basic requirement for health care professionals for research, knowledge, and administrative responsibilities (Oberprieler, Masters, & Gibbs, 2005; Polhamus, Farel & Trester, 2000). Throughout the Case program and particularly the educational leadership track, there are endless opportunities to explore new technologies and information strategies and to seek mentorship with cutting-edge innovations. At graduation I felt equipped with the necessary skills to take leadership positions due to the way these key critical areas were integrated throughout my program.

Graduate outcomes from my DNP program included an increase in scholarly knowledge, improved career prospects, enrichment of research techniques, enhancement of evidence-based practice, and an appreciation and aptitude for technology. The courses added breadth and scope to educational practice and facilitated my development and growth as an educator. The educational preparation has increased my repertoire of creative and innovative strategies, as well as opportunities to sharpen and expand my teaching methodologies. My education throughout the DNP program was meaningful, and mentoring from renowned nurse researchers and educational experts assisted with focusing on relevant and significant nursing issues for research and educational practice.

Many opportunities arose and were created to showcase leadership among the student body. In the program the students were recognized for their experience and leadership in practice and were identified as the experts in practice situations. Development of leadership skills is necessary to ensure successful practice (Bondas, 2006; Cook & Leathard, 2004; Sherman, 2005; Stichler, 2006; Tan, 2006) and is vital to preserve the fundamental nature of nursing within the complex education and health care setting (Bondas, 2006). The educational leadership courses reinforced the strong lifelong learning commitment, the prospect of improving working conditions, ensuring evidence-based curricula, and a duty to the care of the student.

SUMMARY AND FUTURE DIRECTIONS

Nursing is a complex tripartite field encompassing education, research, and practice (Keefe & Pesut, 2004; McKenna, 2005; Moody, Horton-Deutsch, & Pesut, 2006). The debate over the value and appropriateness of the DNP degree diminishes the vital contribution I can make as a DNP graduate to the profession of nursing. I envisage my future as a nurse leader shaping and changing Canadian nursing as it embraces the future. The creation and dissemination of knowledge to my colleagues and/or nursing students is an essential role in the complex health care and education systems. The DNP program at FPB offers a unique, innovative, and balanced approach to managing the distinctness of nursing's tripartite. It focuses on all three aspects, with direct relevance to nursing practice. As an educator I believe the DNP degree provides me with the leadership skills to advance the charge for advocating lifelong learning for all nurses, to ensure that the profession of nursing remains credible and a valuable partner in health care.

REFERENCES

American Association of Colleges of Nursing (AACN). (2004). *AACN position statement on the practice doctorate in nursing.* Retrieved December 12, 2007, from http://www.aacn.nche.edu/DNP/DNPPositionStatement.htm

Bondas, T. (2006). Paths to nursing leadership. *Journal of Nursing Management, 14,* 332–339.

Boyer, E. (1996). Clinical practice as scholarship. *Holistic Nursing Practice, 3,* 1–6.

Bunkers, S. S. (2002). Doctoral education in nursing: Seeking clarity. *Nursing Science Quarterly, 15*(3), 201–208.

Canadian Association of Schools of Nursing (CASN). (2006). *Position statement: Doctoral preparation in nursing.* Retrieved December 12, 2007, from http://www.casn.ca/media.php?mid=203

Canadian Nurses Association (CNA). (2002). *Evidence-based decision-making and nursing practice.* Retrieved December 12, 2007, from http://www.cna-nurses.ca/CNA/documents/pdf/publications/PS63_Evidence_based_Decision_making_Nursing_Practice_e.pdf

Canadian Nurses Association (CNA) & Canadian Association of Schools of Nursing (CASN). (2004). *Joint position statement: Doctoral education in nursing in Canada.* Retrieved December 12, 2007, from http://www.casn.ca/media.php?mid=208

Chandra, A., & Paul III, D. P. (2004). Hospitals' movements toward the electronic medical record: Implications for nurses. *Hospital Topics: Research and Perspectives on Healthcare, 82*(1), 33–36.

Cook, M. J., & Leathard, H. L. (2004). Learning for clinical leadership. *Journal of Nursing Management, 12,* 436–444.

Davis, E. A. (2006). *Toward 2020: Visions for nursing.* Retrieved December 12, 2007, from www.cna-nurses.ca/CNA/documents/pdf/publications/Towards_2020_Snapshot_e.pdf

Doutrich, D., Hoeksel, R., Wykoff, L., & Thiele, J. (2005). Teaching teachers to teach with technology. *The Journal of Continuing Education in Nursing, 36*(1), 25–31.

Frances Payne Bolton School of Nursing. (2007–2008a). *Bulletin: Doctor of nursing practice.* Retrieved December 12, 2007, from http://fpb.case.edu/programs/bulletin.shtm

Frances Payne Bolton School of Nursing. (2007–2008b). *Bulletin: Strategic vision.* Retrieved December 12, 2007, from http://fpb.case.edu/programs/bulletin.shtm

Frances Payne Bolton School of Nursing Centers of Excellence. (n.d.). Retrieved December 12, 2007, from http://fpb.case.edu/Centers/index.shtm

Fulton, J. S., & Lyon, B. L. (2005). The need for some sense making: Doctor of nursing practice. *Online Journal of Issues in Nursing, 10*(3), Manuscript 3. Retrieved December 12, 2007, from http://www.nursingworld.org/ojin

Johnson, J. E. (2001). Thoughts on "e-schooling" for nurse executives (editorial). *Patient Care Management, 17*(1), 2, 11.

Keefe, M. R., & Pesut, D. J. (2004). Appreciative inquiry and leadership transitions. *Journal of Professional Nursing, 20,* 103–109.

Loomis, J. A., Willard, B., & Cohen, J. (2005). Difficult professional choices: Deciding between the PhD and the DNP in nursing. *Online Journal of Issues in Nursing, 10*(3), Manuscript 1. Retrieved December 12, 2007, from http://www.nursingworld.org/ojin

McKenna, H. (2005). Doctoral education: Some treasonable thoughts (editorial). *International Journal of Nursing studies, 42,* 245–246.

Meleis, A. I., & Dracup, K. (2005). The case against the DNP: History, timing, substance, and marginalization. *Online Journal of Issues in Nursing, 10*(3), Manuscript 2. Retrieved December 12, 2007, from http://www.nursingworld.org/ojin

Moody, R. C., Horton-Deutsch, S., & Pesut, D. J. (2006). Appreciative inquiry for leading in complex systems: Supporting the transformation of academic nursing culture. *Journal of Nursing Education, 46*(7), 319–324.

Moore, S. F., Degiorgio, L., Kampfe, C. M., Porter, D. F., Sax, C., McAllan, L., Sales, A. P., & Smith, S. M. (2006). Rehabilitation student perceptions of Web-based learning. *Rehabilitation Education, 20*(1), 31–41.

Oberprieler, G., Masters, K., & Gibbs, T. (2005). Information technology and information literacy for first year health sciences students in South Africa: Matching early and professional needs. *Medical Teacher, 27*(7), 595–598.

O'Sullivan, A. L., Carter, M., Marion, L., Pohl, J. M., & Werner, K. E. (2005). Moving forward together: The practice doctorate in nursing. *Online Journal of Issues in Nursing, 10*(3), Manuscript 4. Retrieved December 12, 2007, from http://www.nursingworld.org/ojin

Pastor, D. K., Cimiotti, J. P., & Stone, P. W. (2004). Doctoral preparation in nursing: What are the options? *Applied Nursing Research, 17*(2), 137–139.

Polhamus, B., Farel, A., & Trester, A. (2000). Enhancing technology skills of maternal and child health professionals. *Maternal and Child Health Journal, 4*(4), 271–275.

Sherman, R. O. (2005). Growing our future nursing leaders. *Nursing Administration Quarterly, 29*(2), 125–132.

Stichler, J. F. (2006). Skills and competencies for today's nurse executive. *AWHONN: The Association of Women's Health, Obstetric and Neonatal Nurses, 10*(3), 255–257.

Tan, P. (2006). Nurturing nursing leadership—Beyond the horizon. *Singapore Nursing Journal, 33*(1), 33–38.

Thorne, S. (2006). Graduate education. In M. McIntyre, E. Thomlinson, & C. McDonald (Eds.), *Realities of Canadian nursing: Professional, practice, and power issues* (2nd ed., pp. 209–226). Philadelphia: Lippincott Williams & Wilkins.

Yam, B. M. C. (2005). Professional doctorate and professional nursing practice. *Nurse Education Today, 25,* 564–572.

12

Voices From the Field: Clinical Nurse Leaders Speak

MEREDITH WALLACE, SANDRA E. FOX, AND PAULA MILLER

The Clinical Nurse Leader (CNL®) is a new role created by the American Association of Colleges of Nursing (AACN) to meet the needs of a failing health care system. CNLs are prepared to function as clinical change agents to improve patient outcomes. Through extensive preparation in leadership, clinical practice, outcomes management and communication, graduates are prepared to improve the health care outcomes of patients in a variety of clinical settings, including acute care and community health settings.

As a new role, it is of great importance to learn from early adopters themselves, namely CNL students. By providing the perspective of recently educated students who are now practicing as CNLs, educators and administrators may build upon current knowledge to expand CNL educational programs and effectively embrace the role of CNLs in the clinical area. The lessons learned from these students may prevent mistakes from being made in the future and provide a framework for future education and clinical frameworks.

The two students who have shared their experiences herein were both post-master's students who were employed at the Tennessee Valley Healthcare System. The Tennessee Healthcare system was the first clinical facility within the Veteran's Administration (VA) system to embrace the CNL role and document the process. Consequently, these students obtained their post-master's education at Vanderbilt University School of Nursing, Tennessee Valley's educational partner. Vanderbilt University School of Nursing worked closely with the American Association of Colleges of nursing and its practice partner to develop a CNL program to improve quality and continuity of care for its environment of interest.

The two students who share their experiences in this chapter discuss their educational program at Vanderbilt and are in agreement that the biggest obstacle within their program was the lack of an available preceptor to instruct them in the CNL roles. This is a problem that has been discussed greatly within the CNL white paper and experienced widely among early adopters. Suggestions for the resolution of this problem include the facilitation of a clinical experience with nursing experts with great exposure to other health care system departments, including pharmacy, risk management, patient safety, finance, and quality assurance (Rusch, 2006).

A great contribution of this chapter is that the students share early clinically innovative work. The first student conducted a series of clinical projects on improving outcomes of surgical patients, postoperatively. As can be seen from her experience, the CNL role resulted in positive patient outcomes in terms of decreases in transfusion rates and flexion contractures. Interestingly, the evaluation process that is such an integral part of the CNL educational program resulted in a further assessment and refined protocol, which resulted in improved infection rates on the CNL graduate's unit. The second student focused her early clinical energy on reducing the no-show rates of gastrointestinal (GI) clients at the procedure lab. Her successful project, resulted in a decrease in the no-show rates from 30% down to 16% over the project period. Clearly, the CNL outcomes resulted in improved staff and patient satisfaction, as well as decreased costs to the health care facility.

The CNL role is new and has the potential to greatly improve the health care system. As seen in the experiences of these new CNL graduates, patient and system outcomes are diverse, but consistently positive. The CNL role is an exciting addition to clinical practice from multiple perspectives. The following excerpts detail the experiences of these new graduates, illustrating the CNL possibilities for promoting outcomes for the nursing profession and health care system, as well as positive outcomes for patients.

EDUCATION PROGRAM AND CLINICAL PRACTICE PERSPECTIVES: SANDRA E. FOX

The clinical nurse leader (CNL) inpatient role at Tennessee Valley Healthcare System was transitioned from a case management/discharge planner role. The goal was to increase the involvement in the clinical practice on the ward by assessing the current patient care outcomes. After the outcomes were assessed and analyzed, the CNL coordinated lateral integration of the pertinent disciplines to develop interdisciplinary plans to improve the patient care outcomes. Our chief nurse encouraged us to enter the Clinical Management Post-Master's Certificate program offered by Vanderbilt University, which would satisfy the requirements for certification offered by the American Association of Colleges of Nursing.

The curriculum included advanced pathophysiology and pharmacology, program development, and health care assessment. These clinical courses helped us to develop our clinical assessment skills and program development to a more complex level of patient care. These classes provided us a framework to begin to organize our initial needs assessments and develop microsystem changes needed in our assigned clinical areas. Our clinical experiences enabled us to compare the systems at other facilities with the systems in which we currently operated.

One inherent weakness that was impossible to avoid was that there were no other clinical nurse leaders at that time to collaborate with and provide clinical experiences across the patient care spectrum. We were truly pioneers, developing the role as we applied the educational resources to the needs we identified. We were not only building careers but educating other staff about our roles and trying to maintain a clear definition of what we were responsible for, not only for ourselves, but to those we were in contact with.

A true strength of the clinical education experience at Vanderbilt University was that it allowed us to incorporate our classroom education directly into our daily work assignments. In other words, we were allowed to use our clinical time to design our roles working with our clinical advisors in our current work environment. This enabled us to develop and implement our needs assessments and plans of care, applying the classroom expertise we gained from our instructors. Incorporating the teaching and learning theories we had just learned in the classroom into our daily practice, we designed patient care microsystems and redesigned educational processes that helped us to achieve our desired outcomes. This was invaluable as we developed new microsystems of nursing care that further set us apart from a staff nurse role to an advanced generalist role.

My first assignment as a surgical CNL was to organize the discharge planning role on a busy 32-bed surgical ward. My first few months as an acting clinical nurse leader (certification had not yet been developed) were spent learning and implementing the discharge planning process. The surgical ward at our facility cares for all of the surgical specialties, and patients having different surgeries, of course, have different discharge needs. Orthopedic patients often need post-discharge physical therapy. New tracheostomy patients need intensive teaching, suction equipment, and many types of supplies. Home health nurses followed many patients upon discharge and often changed dressings or administered IV antibiotics via peripherally inserted central catheter (PICC) lines. All of these issues required an assessment of the patient's and significant others' abilities, ordering supplies and equipment, and coordinating the various outpatient services. There were also many details to attend to with transfers to rehabilitation and long-term care facilities.

Another one of my responsibilities was to focus on the surgical outcomes of our most frequently performed major surgeries. Our unit provided nursing care for approximately 100 patients per year who underwent total knee arthroplasty. A chart review to determine the rates of complications for the last year was completed as part of my needs assessment. Complications identified included flexion contracture, overdose, and infection. A literature review was also completed, and an interdisciplinary group including staff nurses, physical therapists, orthopedic surgeons, and me met to develop protocols to address these issues. Nursing interventions included a change in patient positioning with a pillow under the ankle to increase leg extension, and more intensive focus on the importance of extension of the operative joint by physical therapy and the nursing staff. Patients and family were instructed to have only the patients operate the administration of patient-controlled analgesia, and, as the clinical nurse leader, I monitored the type and dose of analgesics ordered in relation to the age, weight and medical history of the patient. Many elderly patients react very strongly to narcotic analgesics, particularly if they are not accustomed to taking analgesics as outpatients.

During the needs assessment I noted that patients were transfused based on widely varying lab results independent of any symptomatology.

The literature noted that there is a transient immunosuppression after transfusion, and, after discussion with the orthopedic team, it was agreed that patients would not be transfused unless the hematocrit was below 23 or the patient was symptomatic with orthostatic hypotension, dizziness, or weakness with ambulation. Other interventions included a preoperative prep with intranasal mupirocin for 5 days preoperatively, with a chlorhexidine shower the day prior to surgery. These measures have been shown to markedly decrease the incidence of Methicillin-resistant *Staphylococcus aureus* (MRSA) infection in orthopedic surgery. The protocol also included cleaning the incision with hydrogen peroxide and applying a telfa-island pad to protect incisional staples from trauma or contamination. The patients were instructed in the application of the dressing, and supplies were ordered upon discharge.

After a year of protocol implementation there were significant decreases in transfusion rates and flexion contractures. The infection rate, however, had gone up. The protocol was reassessed, and we began to remove foley catheters while the patients were still on their perioperative antibiotics. The infection rate subsequently decreased.

Next I began to develop protocols for hip replacement surgery and colon surgery with those disciplines. I was also working with our Informational Resource Management team to develop electronic order sets to allow a more consistent implementation of the protocols. As a teaching facility, our surgical residents rotate, and it is difficult to have consistent postoperative orders.

Our administrative team identified a problem that they felt needed to be a priority, surgical cancellations. I was then moved to the perioperative setting and began a new needs assessment. The ambulatory surgery staff confirmed surgeries after the surgical schedule was finalized. The schedule was finalized by 11:00 A.M. the day prior to the procedure. Patients who called that afternoon who for various reasons could not have surgery the next morning were thus cancellations. Administration requested that I do what could be done to immediately make a change in the situation, so I took over confirming the surgeries, but did so as early as possible. Our anesthesia department requires that metformin and olanzepine be held for 48 hours preoperatively to prevent malignant hyperthermia as a complication of general anesthesia. Depending upon the type of surgery the patient is having, anticoagulants and platelet aggregation inhibitors need to be held for varying lengths of time. Most neurosurgeries, urologic surgeries, and many ear-nose-throat surgeries require anticoagulants, aspirin and other nonsteroidal anti-inflammatory medications, vitamin E, and garlic supplements be held for 5 to 10 days preoperatively. Stopping these medications may be the judgment of the surgeon, or other disciplines such as cardiology may be consulted. Some patients require transition from Coumadin (warfarin) to a low-molecular-weight heparin such as lovenox subcutaneously, which can be held the night before and the morning of surgery. These issues were not being addressed regularly by the residents and were not the responsibility of anesthesiology. Therefore, when a patient was "boarded" for surgery the morning prior, these issues had often not been addressed.

An interdisciplinary task force met to identify issues that were obstructions to the surgical process. This team consisted of staff nurses, a computer technician, administrative nursing staff, a Veterans Integrated Service Networks (VISN) leader, the director of the dental department, who participated in problem solving in many facilities throughout the VA system. We developed a flowchart and worked through several issues with the Primary Care Group, Anesthesiology, and Surgery departments. Issues such as uncontrolled hypertension and diabetes must be optimally managed before referral to a surgical specialty for elective procedures. The task force group proposed centralizing the surgery scheduling and finalizing the surgical schedule 48 hours before the surgery instead of less than 24 hours to allow more time to resolve issues that may result in surgery cancellations. A PowerPoint presentation was made to senior management. During our past fiscal year the Nashville VA Medical Center has undergone significant administrative changes. As the clinical nurse leader in the preoperative evaluation center, operating room, and recovery room, I continued to make efforts to minimize surgery cancellations in the areas I was able to influence. I also developed clinical skills in preoperative evaluation and post-anesthesia recovery so I could assist staff in those areas. My operating room experiences were mostly observation, as developing proficiency in scrubbing and circulating takes several months of intensive orientation.

At the end of fiscal year 2007 I evaluated the impact my interventions had had on the surgery cancellation rate. The figures I used to calculate changes were kept by the computer technician in the surgery service and were not statistics I collected. During that year there was a decrease in "patient related reasons for cancellations" of 55%! These results were shared with the surgery service, senior administration, and a doctoral student with whom I had collaborated. The cancellation results have been presented in an abstract that I wrote for the AACN CNL Conference in January of 2008. Senior administration and the head of surgery then decided to go ahead with the plan to centralize surgery scheduling and require that elective surgeries be scheduled at least 48 hours preoperatively. When a service does not schedule their cases in time, other services are offering their block time. The first week this was implemented there was a 25% increase in operating room utilization.

TRANSITION TO THE PROFESSIONAL ROLE AND CLINICAL SUCCESS: PAULA MILLER

My position was as a CNL in an outpatient endoscopy procedure lab. The outpatient CNL role was being closely evaluated at this time and I was consistently observed by my nurse executives to validate a need for this role in the outpatient setting. I firmly believed this role was needed, as I watched daily the benefits of the microsystem changes that were implemented. One of my major outcomes was a decrease in the no-show cancellation rate in our GI procedure lab. Patients were coming unprepared physically and emotionally for the procedures they were about to experience. As a clinical nurse leader, my initial assessment indicated that patient needs in scheduling were in conflict with current scheduling strategies and there was a great need to improve in education and communication with patients. This applied not only to the nursing staff but to the clerical staff as well.

Collaborating with the chief gastroenterologist of our lab, we adopted the evidence-based practice principles of Advance Clinic Access into our clinical lab. Working with these principles, we developed microsystem process changes, and, in collaboration with the nurse manager, we implemented these changes with the nursing staff. Outcomes came quickly, as our no-show cancellation rates were cut in half from 30% in 2004 and 28% in 2005 to 14% in 2006 and 16% in 2007. Patient satisfaction increased as patients were processed through procedures quickly, and any delay we had in their care we could identify as a direct result of unpredictable staffing shortages and not the microsystem process itself.

Some examples of microsystem process changes were the implementation of a more efficient scheduling process, which led to the changes in the functioning of our recovery room, and the creation of a preprocedure prep station. These two process changes allowed us to increase our patient load by 50 to 75 patients per month with no increase in supplies or personnel. Staff satisfaction increased as well as patient satisfaction, as staff became more vested in their work. Predictable workloads allowed the staff to plan their workloads more efficiently, and the nurse manager was able to allow for planned days off without affecting patient care thereby, promoting staff satisfaction and retention. Staff performance also improved as staff began to work on professional goals, such as working on research, which led to article publication in professional nursing journals and magazines. They also worked with the CNL to update existing policies that affected the endoscopy lab that were no longer meeting patient care needs. Nursing staff also became the model for the facility for implementing new processes such as the Time-Out process, creating a Time-Out educational CD, along with a computer charting form that is currently being planned for hospital-wide use. The AACN became interested in our accomplishments as we joined them to create educational CDs describing the creation of the Clinical Nurse Leader role at our facility. These CDs are in demand nationwide, as is our expertise in development of the CNL role. The clinical nurse leaders at Tennessee Valley are contacted routinely by e-mail from students and executives all over the United States in an effort to gain insight into how they are structuring their roles and implementing process improvement projects.

An immense barrier encountered was a lack of understanding of the Clinical Nurse Leader role. Resistance to change was seen not only by the staff nurses but by the medical staff and nursing management staff encountered by the clinical nurse leaders. Nurse executives became facilitators of the role and provided support and education to the physicians and other executive leaders in direct contact with the CNL. The chief of staff has been an important role supporter and has chosen to use the CNL as a key player in maximizing the efficiency of our operating room to better meet our veterans' needs. The assistant chief of medical service, who is also in charge of the endoscopy department, is a strong supporter of the CNL role, as changes made by the endoscopy CNL in the procedure lab included full support of the physicians on staff.

The most important facilitator of the CNL role has been promoting the outcomes we have achieved. Getting patient care outcome information to the appropriate members of our team and to the patients as well has been vital in keeping the role active at our facility. It has been imperative to have the nurse executive team in full support as we both developed our roles. Their promotion of the CNL role while in direct contact with staff, nursing management, and physicians as well has been essential to the successes we have enjoyed. Future endeavors or responsibilities for the CNL in the endoscopy lab are growing steadily, as projects in fecal occult blood test monitoring, capsule endoscopy, and monitoring of fee-based screening colonoscopy patients are being case-managed by the CNL, resulting in more efficient and cost-effective patient care.

Being a master's-prepared nurse is essential to becoming a clinical nurse leader. Advanced nursing and clinical management knowledge gained at the master's level of education is vital to role success. Academic and clinical knowledge gained in preparation for the master's level of education cannot be replaced, as the patients of today have complex medical and psychosocial needs. These needs demand nurse experts who are not only trained in complex nursing care, but also in macrosystem and microsytem patient care management, while incorporating community resource management as well.

Our educational preparation has taught us system development theories and complex patient care approaches to allow us to assess and develop plans to manage the unique and complex needs of the veteran patient. We anticipate continuing our education to the doctoral level, as we are finding that having more knowledge about research and development is essential at the clinical level.

SUMMARY AND FUTURE DIRECTIONS

We see the Clinical Nurse Leader role as satisfying the health care system's need for a change agent to identify not only the complex needs of today's patient but to do this in a cost-effective and efficient manner that is vital to the future of today's health care. As the complexity of health care continues to escalate, it is necessary to have someone charged with organizing and coordinating all of the many components. The organization and coordination of health care needs require a great deal of clinical expertise as well as educational and interpersonal communication skills.

The areas in which we have implemented the roles were initially approached performing a comprehensive needs assessment. Patient outcomes and access to care are important components of the needs assessment. As practicing CNLs we have come to recognize that a needs assessment is an ongoing process to be redeveloped with health care management at different levels as the patient's needs change. For example, after the needs assessment and lateral integration of knowledge from another professional, such as a clinical nurse specialist, a plan of care can be changed and implemented by the CNL. Outcomes are then measured, and the plan, protocol, or microsystem is analyzed and changed accordingly to satisfy the efficiency of patient care provided.

We believe the need for this role will continue to grow as the complexity of health care technology advances, forcing a need for more complex patient care and education. Patients today demand more knowledge as they are faced with making more complex decisions in their plan of care.

REFERENCE

Rusch, L. (2006). *The CNL® pilot at Hunterdon Medical Center.* Presentation given at AACN Regional Conferences on Clinical Nurse Leader, Denver, CO, June, 2006.

Appendix A

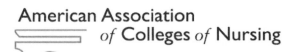

American Association *of* Colleges *of* Nursing

ADVANCING HIGHER EDUCATION IN NURSING

One Dupont Circle NW, Suite 530 ·Washington, DC 20036 · 202-463-6930 tel · 202-785-8320 fax · www.aacn.nche.edu

The Essentials of Doctoral Education for Advanced Nursing

TABLE OF CONTENTS

INTRODUCTION

Background

Doctoral programs in nursing fall into two principal types: research-focused and practice-focused. Most research-focused programs grant the Doctor of Philosophy degree (PhD), while a small percentage offers the Doctor of Nursing Science degree (DNS, DSN, or DNSc). Designed to prepare nurse scientists and scholars, these programs focus heavily on scientific content and research methodology; and all require an original research project and the completion and defense of a dissertation or linked research papers. Practice-focused doctoral programs are designed to prepare experts in specialized advanced nursing practice. They focus heavily on practice that is innovative and evidence-based, reflecting the application of credible research findings. The two types of doctoral programs differ in their goals and the competencies of their graduates. They represent complementary, alternative approaches to the highest level of educational preparation in nursing.

The concept of a practice doctorate in nursing is not new. However, this course of study has evolved considerably over the 20 years since the first practice-focused nursing doctorate, the Doctor of Nursing (ND), was initiated as an entry-level degree. Because research- and practice-focused programs are distinctly different, the current position of the American Association of Colleges of Nursing (AACN, 2004) [detailed in the Position Statement on the Practice Doctorate in Nursing] is that: "The two types of doctorates, research-focused and practice-focused, may coexist within the same education unit" and that the practice-focused degree should be the Doctor of Nursing Practice (DNP). Recognizing the need for consistency in the degrees required for advanced nursing practice, all existing ND programs have transitioned to the DNP.

Comparison Between Research-Focused and Practice-Focused Doctoral Education

Research- and practice-focused doctoral programs in nursing share rigorous and demanding expectations: a scholarly approach to the discipline, and a commitment to the advancement of the profession. Both are terminal degrees in the discipline, one in practice and one in research. However, there are distinct differences between the two degree programs. For example, practice-focused programs understandably place greater emphasis on practice, and less emphasis on theory, meta-theory, research methodology, and statistics than is apparent in research-focused programs. Whereas all research-focused programs require an extensive research study that is reported in a dissertation or through the development of linked research papers, practice-focused doctoral programs generally include integrative practice experiences and an intense practice immersion experience. Rather than a knowledge-generating research effort, the student in a practice-focused program generally carries out a practice application–oriented "final DNP project," which is an integral part of the integrative practice experience.

AACN Task Force on the Practice Doctorate in Nursing

The AACN Task Force to Revise Quality Indicators for Doctoral Education found that the Indicators of Quality in Research-Focused Doctoral Programs in Nursing are applicable to doctoral programs leading to a PhD or a DNS degree (AACN, 2001b, p. 1). Therefore, practice-focused doctoral programs will need to be examined separately from research-focused programs. This finding, coupled with the growing interest in practice doctorates prompted the establishment of the AACN Task Force on the Practice Doctorate in Nursing in 2002. This task force was convened to examine trends in practice-focused doctoral education and make recommendations about the need for and nature of such programs in nursing. Task force members included representatives from universities that already offered or were planning to offer the practice doctorate, from universities that offered only the research doctorate in nursing, from a specialty professional organization, and from nursing service administration. The task force was charged to describe patterns in existing practice-focused doctoral programs; clarify the purpose of the practice doctorate, particularly as differentiated from the research doctorate; identify preferred goals, titles, and tracks; and identify and make recommendations about key issues. Over a two-year period, this task force adopted an inclusive approach that included: (a) securing information from multiple sources about existing programs, trends, and potential benefits of a practice doctorate; (b) providing multiple opportunities for open discussion of related issues at AACN and other professional meetings; and (c) subjecting draft recommendations to discussion and input from multiple stakeholder groups. The final position statement was approved by the AACN Board of Directors in March 2004 and subsequently adopted by the membership.

The 2004 DNP position statement calls for a transformational change in the education required for professional nurses who will practice at the most advanced level of nursing. The recommendation that nurses practicing at the highest level should receive doctoral-level preparation emerged from multiple factors, including the expansion of scientific knowledge required for safe nursing practice and growing concerns regarding the quality of patient care delivery and outcomes. Practice demands associated with an increasingly complex health care system created a mandate for reassessing the education for clinical practice for all health professionals, including nurses.

A significant component of the work by the task force that developed the 2004 position statement was the development of a definition that described the scope of advanced nursing practice. Advanced nursing practice is broadly defined by AACN (2004) as:

> *any form of nursing intervention that influences health care outcomes for individuals or populations, including the direct care of individual patients, management of care for individuals and populations, administration of nursing and health care organizations, and the development and implementation of health policy.* (p. 2)

Furthermore, the DNP position statement (AACN, 2004, p. 4) identifies the benefits of practice-focused doctoral programs as:

- Development of needed advanced competencies for increasingly complex practice, faculty, and leadership roles;
- Enhanced knowledge to improve nursing practice and patient outcomes;
- Enhanced leadership skills to strengthen practice and health care delivery;
- Better match of program requirements and credits and time with the credential earned;
- Provision of an advanced educational credential for those who require advanced practice knowledge but do not need or want a strong research focus (e.g., practice faculty);
- Enhanced ability to attract individuals to nursing from non-nursing backgrounds; and
- Increased supply of faculty for practice instruction.

As a result of the membership vote to adopt the recommendation that the nursing profession establish the DNP as its highest practice degree, the AACN Board of Directors, in January 2005, created the Task Force on the Essentials of Nursing Education for the Doctorate of Nursing Practice and charged this task force with development of the curricular expectations that will guide and shape DNP education.

The DNP Essentials Task Force is comprised of individuals representing multiple constituencies in advanced nursing practice (see Appendix B). The task force conducted regional hearings from September 2005 to January 2006 to provide opportunities for feedback from a diverse group of stakeholders. These hearings were designed using an iterative process to develop this document. In total, 620 participants representing 231 educational institutions and a wide variety of professional organizations participated in the regional meetings. Additionally, a national stakeholders' conference was held in October 2005 in which 65 leaders from 45 professional organizations participated.

Context of Graduate Education in Nursing

Graduate education in nursing occurs within the context of societal demands and needs as well as the interprofessional work environment. The Institute of Medicine (IOM, 2003) and the National Research Council of the National Academies (2005, p. 74) have called for nursing education that prepares individuals for practice with interdisciplinary, information systems, quality improvement, and patient safety expertise.

In hallmark reports, the IOM (1999, 2001, 2003) has focused attention on the state of health care delivery, patient safety issues, health professions education, and leadership for nursing practice. These reports highlight the human errors and financial burden caused by fragmentation and system failures in health care. In addition, the IOM calls for dramatic restructuring of all health professionals' education. Among the recommendations resulting from these reports are that health care organizations and groups promote health care that is safe, effective, client-centered, timely, efficient, and equitable; that health professionals should be educated to deliver patient-centered care as members of an interdisciplinary team, emphasizing evidence-based practice, quality improvement, and informatics; and, that the best-prepared senior level nurses should be in key leadership positions and participating in executive decisions.

Since AACN published *The Essentials of Master's Education for Advanced Practice Nursing* in 1996 and the first set of indicators for quality doctoral nursing education in 1986, several trends in health professional education and health care delivery have emerged. Over the past two decades, graduate programs in nursing have expanded from 220 institutions offering 39 doctoral programs and 180 master's programs in 1986 to 518 institutions offering 101 doctoral programs and 417 master's programs in 2006. Increasing numbers of these programs offer preparation for certification in advanced practice specialty roles such as nurse practitioners, nurse midwives, nurse anesthetists, and clinical nurse specialists. Specialization is also a trend in other health professional education. During this same time period, the explosion in information, technology, and new scientific evidence to guide practice has extended the length of educational programs in nursing and the other health professions. In response to these trends, several other health professions such as pharmacy, physical therapy, occupational therapy, and audiology have moved to the professional or practice doctorate for entry into these respective professions.

Further, support for doctoral education for nursing practice was found in a review of current master's level nursing programs (AACN, 2004, p. 4). This review indicated that many programs already have expanded significantly in response to the above concerns, creating curricula that exceed the usual credit load and duration for a typical master's degree. The expansion of credit requirements in these programs beyond the norm for a master's degree raises additional concerns that professional nurse graduates are not receiving the appropriate degree for a very complex and demanding academic experience. Many of these programs, in reality, require a program of study closer to the curricular expectations for other professional doctoral programs rather than for master's level study.

Relationships of Master's, Practice Doctorate, and Research Doctorate Programs

The master's degree (MSN) historically has been the degree for specialized advanced nursing practice. With development of DNP programs, this new degree will become the preferred preparation for specialty nursing practice. As educational institutions transition from the master's to DNP degree for advanced practice specialty preparation, a variety of program articulations and pathways are planned. One constant is true for all of these models. The DNP is a graduate degree and is built upon the generalist foundation acquired through a baccalaureate or advanced generalist master's in nursing. The *Essentials of Baccalaureate Education*

(AACN, 1998) summarizes the core knowledge and competencies of the baccalaureate-prepared nurse. Building on this foundation, the DNP core competencies establish a base for advanced nursing practice in an area of specialization. Ultimately, the terminal degree options in nursing will fall into two primary education pathways: professional entry degree (baccalaureate or master's) to DNP degree or professional entry degree (baccalaureate or master's) to PhD degree. As in other disciplines with practice doctorates, some individuals may choose to combine a DNP with a PhD.

Regardless of the entry point, DNP curricula are designed so that all students attain DNP end-of-program competencies. Because different entry points exist, the curricula must be individualized for candidates based on their prior education and experience. For example, early in the transition period, many students entering DNP programs will have a master's degree that has been built on AACN's *Master's Essentials*. Graduates of such programs would already have attained many of the competencies defined in the *DNP Essentials*. Therefore, their program will be designed to provide those DNP competencies not previously attained. If a candidate is entering the program with a non-nursing baccalaureate degree, his/her program of study likely will be longer than for a candidate entering the program with a baccalaureate or master's in nursing. While specialty advanced nursing education will be provided at the doctoral level in DNP programs, new options for advanced generalist master's education are being developed.

DNP Graduates and Academic Roles

Nursing as a practice profession requires both practice experts and nurse scientists to expand the scientific basis for patient care. Doctoral education in nursing is designed to prepare nurses for the highest level of leadership in practice and scientific inquiry. The DNP is a degree designed specifically to prepare individuals for specialized nursing practice, and *The Essentials of Doctoral Education for Advanced Nursing Practice* articulates the competencies for all nurses practicing at this level.

In some instances, individuals who acquire the DNP will seek to fill roles as educators and will use their considerable practice expertise to educate the next generation of nurses. As in other disciplines (e.g., engineering, business, law), the major focus of the educational program must be on the area of practice specialization within the discipline, not the process of teaching. However, individuals who desire a role as an educator, whether that role is operationalized in a practice environment or the academy, should have additional preparation in the science of pedagogy to augment their ability to transmit the science of the profession they practice and teach. This additional preparation may occur in formal course work during the DNP program.

Some teaching strategies and learning principles will be incorporated into the DNP curriculum as it relates to patient education. However, the basic DNP curriculum does not prepare the graduate for a faculty teaching role any more than the PhD curriculum does. Graduates of either program planning a faculty career will need preparation in teaching methodologies, curriculum design and development, and program evaluation. This preparation is in addition to that required for their area of specialized nursing practice or research in the case of the PhD graduate.

THE ESSENTIALS OF DOCTORAL EDUCATION FOR ADVANCED NURSING PRACTICE

The following *DNP Essentials* outline the curricular elements and competencies that must be present in programs conferring the Doctor of Nursing Practice degree. The DNP is a degree title, like the PhD or MSN, and does not designate in what specialty a graduate is prepared. DNP graduates will be prepared for a variety of nursing practice roles. The *DNP Essentials* delineated here address the foundational competencies that are core to all advanced nursing practice roles. However, the depth and focus of the core competencies will vary based on the particular role for which the student is preparing. For example, students preparing for organizational leadership or administrative roles will have increased depth in organizational and systems leadership; those preparing for policy roles will have increased depth in health care policy; and those preparing for APRN roles (nurse practitioners, clinical nurse specialists, nurse anesthetists, and nurse midwives) will have more specialized content in an area of advanced practice nursing.

Additionally, it is important to understand that the delineation of these competencies should not be interpreted to mean that a separate course for each of the *DNP Essentials* should be offered. Curricula will differ in emphases based on the particular specialties for which students are being prepared.

The DNP curriculum is conceptualized as having two components:

1   DNP Essentials 1 through 8 are the foundational outcome competencies deemed essential for all graduates of a DNP program regardless of specialty or functional focus.

2   Specialty competencies/content prepare the DNP graduate for those practice and didactic learning experiences for a particular specialty. **Competencies, content, and practica experiences needed for specific roles in specialty areas are delineated by national specialty nursing organizations.**

The *DNP Essentials* document outlines and defines the eight foundational Essentials and provides some introductory comments on specialty competencies/content. The specialized content, as defined by specialty organizations, complements the areas of core content defined by the *DNP Essentials* and constitutes the major component of DNP programs. DNP curricula should include these two components as appropriate to the specific advanced nursing practice specialist being prepared. Additionally, the faculty of each DNP program has the academic freedom to create innovative and integrated curricula to meet the competencies outlined in the *Essentials* document.

Essential I: Scientific Underpinnings for Practice

The practice doctorate in nursing provides the terminal academic preparation for nursing practice. The scientific underpinnings of this education reflect the complexity of practice at the doctoral level and the rich heritage that is the conceptual foundation of nursing. The discipline of nursing is focused on:

- The principles and laws that govern the life-process, well-being, and optimal function of human beings, sick or well;
- The patterning of human behavior in interaction with the environment in normal life events and critical life situations;
- The nursing actions or processes by which positive changes in health status are affected; and
- The wholeness or health of human beings recognizing that they are in continuous interaction with their environments (Donaldson & Crowley, 1978; Fawcett, 2005; Gortner, 1980).

DNP graduates possess a wide array of knowledge gleaned from the sciences and have the ability to translate that knowledge quickly and effectively to benefit patients in the daily demands of practice environments (Porter-O'Grady, 2003). Preparation to address current and future practice issues requires a strong scientific foundation for practice.

The scientific foundation of nursing practice has expanded and includes a focus on both the natural and social sciences. These sciences that provide a foundation for nursing practice include human biology, genomics, the science of therapeutics, the psychosocial sciences, as well as the science of complex organizational structures. In addition, philosophical, ethical, and historical issues inherent in the development of science create a context for the application of the natural and social sciences. Nursing science also has created a significant body of knowledge to guide nursing practice and has expanded the scientific underpinnings of the discipline. Nursing science frames the development of middle range theories and concepts to guide nursing practice. Advances in the foundational and nursing sciences will occur continuously, and nursing curricula must remain sensitive to emerging and new scientific findings to prepare the DNP for evolving practice realities.

The DNP program prepares the graduate to:

1   Integrate nursing science with knowledge from ethics, the biophysical, psychosocial, analytical, and organizational sciences as the basis for the highest level of nursing practice.
2   Use science-based theories and concepts to:
   ■ Determine the nature and significance of health and health care delivery phenomena;
   ■ Describe the actions and advanced strategies to enhance, alleviate, and ameliorate health and health care delivery phenomena as appropriate; and
   ■ Evaluate outcomes.
3   Develop and evaluate new practice approaches based on nursing theories and theories from other disciplines.

Essential II: Organizational and Systems Leadership for Quality Improvement and Systems Thinking

Organizational and systems leadership are critical for DNP graduates to improve patient and health care outcomes. Doctoral level knowledge and skills in these areas are consistent with nursing and health care goals to eliminate health disparities and to promote patient safety and excellence in practice.

DNP graduates' practice includes not only direct care but also a focus on the needs of a panel of patients, a target population, a set of populations, or a broad community. These graduates are distinguished by their abilities to conceptualize new care delivery models that are based in contemporary nursing science and that are feasible within current organizational, political, cultural, and economic perspectives.

Graduates must be skilled in working within organizational and policy arenas and in the actual provision of patient care by themselves and/or others. For example, DNP graduates must understand principles of practice management, including conceptual and practical strategies for balancing productivity with quality of care. They must be able to assess the impact of practice policies and procedures on meeting the health needs of the patient populations with whom they practice. DNP graduates must be proficient in quality improvement strategies and in creating and sustaining changes at the organizational and policy levels. Improvements in practice are neither sustainable nor measurable without corresponding changes in organizational arrangements, organizational and professional culture, and the financial structures to support practice. DNP graduates have the ability to evaluate the cost effectiveness of care and use principles of economics and finance to redesign effective and realistic care delivery strategies. In addition, DNP graduates have the ability to organize care to address emerging practice problems and the ethical dilemmas that emerge as new diagnostic and therapeutic technologies evolve. Accordingly, DNP graduates are able to assess risk and collaborate with others to manage risks ethically, based on professional standards.

Thus, advanced nursing practice includes an organizational and systems leadership component that emphasizes practice, ongoing improvement of health outcomes, and ensuring patient safety. In each case, nurses should be prepared with sophisticated expertise in assessing organizations, identifying systems issues, and facilitating organization-wide changes in practice delivery. In addition, advanced nursing practice requires political skills, systems thinking, and the business and financial acumen needed for the analysis of practice quality and costs.

The DNP program prepares the graduate to:

1 Develop and evaluate care delivery approaches that meet current and future needs of patient populations based on scientific findings in nursing and other clinical sciences, as well as organizational, political, and economic sciences.
2 Ensure accountability for quality of health care and patient safety for populations with whom they work.

a Use advanced communication skills/processes to lead quality improvement and patient safety initiatives in health care systems.

b Employ principles of business, finance, economics, and health policy to develop and implement effective plans for practice-level and/or system-wide practice initiatives that will improve the quality of care delivery.

c Develop and/or monitor budgets for practice initiatives.

d Analyze the cost-effectiveness of practice initiatives accounting for risk and improvement of health care outcomes.

e Demonstrate sensitivity to diverse organizational cultures and populations, including patients and providers.

3 Develop and/or evaluate effective strategies for managing the ethical dilemmas inherent in patient care, the health care organization, and research.

Essential III: Clinical Scholarship and Analytical Methods for Evidence-Based Practice

Scholarship and research are the hallmarks of doctoral education. Although basic research has been viewed as the first and most essential form of scholarly activity, an enlarged perspective of scholarship has emerged through alternative paradigms that involve more than discovery of new knowledge (Boyer, 1990). These paradigms recognize that (a) the scholarship of discovery and integration "reflects the investigative and synthesizing traditions of academic life" (Boyer, p. 21); (b) scholars give meaning to isolated facts and make connections across disciplines through the scholarship of integration; and (c) the scholar applies knowledge to solve a problem via the scholarship of application (referred to as the scholarship of practice in nursing). This application involves the translation of research into practice and the dissemination and integration of new knowledge, which are key activities of DNP graduates. The scholarship of application expands the realm of knowledge beyond mere discovery and directs it toward humane ends. Nursing practice epitomizes the scholarship of application through its position where the sciences, human caring, and human needs meet and new understandings emerge.

Nurses have long recognized that scholarly nursing practice is characterized by the discovery of new phenomena and the application of new discoveries in increasingly complex practice situations. The integration of knowledge from diverse sources and across disciplines, and the application of knowledge to solve practice problems and improve health outcomes are only two of the many ways new phenomena and knowledge are generated other than through research (AACN, 1999; Diers, 1995; Palmer, 1986; Sigma Theta Tau International, 1999). Research-focused doctoral programs in nursing are designed to prepare graduates with the research skills necessary for discovering new knowledge in the discipline. In contrast, DNP graduates engage in advanced nursing practice and provide leadership for evidence-based practice. This requires competence in knowledge application activities: the translation of research in practice, the evaluation of practice, improvement of the reliability of health care practice and outcomes, and participation in collaborative research (DePalma & McGuire, 2005). Therefore, DNP programs focus on the translation of new science, and its application and evaluation. In addition, DNP graduates generate evidence through their practice to guide improvements in practice and outcomes of care.

The DNP program prepares the graduate to:

1   Use analytic methods to critically appraise existing literature and other evidence to determine and implement the best evidence for practice.

2   Design and implement processes to evaluate outcomes of practice, practice patterns, and systems of care within a practice setting, health care organization, or community against national benchmarks to determine variances in practice outcomes and population trends.

3   Design, direct, and evaluate quality improvement methodologies to promote safe, timely, effective, efficient, equitable, and patient-centered care.

4   Apply relevant findings to develop practice guidelines and improve practice and the practice environment.

5   Use information technology and research methods appropriately to:

- Collect appropriate and accurate data to generate evidence for nursing practice
- Inform and guide the design of databases that generate meaningful evidence for nursing practice
- Analyze data from practice
- Design evidence-based interventions

■ Predict and analyze outcomes
■ Examine patterns of behavior and outcomes
■ Identify gaps in evidence for practice

6 Function as a practice specialist/consultant in collaborative knowledge-generating research.
7 Disseminate findings from evidence-based practice and research to improve health care outcomes.

Essential IV: Information Systems/Technology and Patient Care Technology for the Improvement and Transformation of Health Care

DNP graduates are distinguished by their abilities to use information systems/technology to support and improve patient care and health care systems and provide leadership within health care systems and/or academic settings. Knowledge and skills related to information systems/technology and patient care technology prepare the DNP graduate to apply new knowledge, manage individual and aggregate level information, and assess the efficacy of patient care technology appropriate to a specialized area of practice. DNP graduates also design, select, and use information systems/technology to evaluate programs of care, outcomes of care, and care systems. Information systems/technology provide a mechanism to apply budget and productivity tools, practice information systems and decision supports, and Web-based learning or intervention tools to support and improve patient care.

DNP graduates must also be proficient in the use of information systems/technology resources to implement quality improvement initiatives and support practice and administrative decision making. Graduates must demonstrate knowledge of standards and principles for selecting and evaluating information systems and patient care technology, and related ethical, regulatory, and legal issues.

The DNP program prepares the graduate to:

1 Design, select, use, and evaluate programs that evaluate and monitor outcomes of care, care systems, and quality improvement including, consumer use of health care information systems.
2 Analyze and communicate critical elements necessary to the selection, use, and evaluation of health care information systems and patient care technology.

3 Demonstrate the conceptual ability and technical skills to develop and execute an evaluation plan involving data extraction
from practice information systems and databases.

4 Provide leadership in the evaluation and resolution of ethical
and legal issues within health care systems relating to the use of
information, information technology, communication networks,
and patient care technology.

5 Evaluate consumer health information sources for accuracy,
timeliness, and appropriateness.

Essential V: Health Care Policy for Advocacy in Health Care

Health care policy—whether it is created through governmental actions, institutional decision making, or organizational standards—creates
a framework that can facilitate or impede the delivery of health care
services or the ability of the provider to engage in practice to address
health care needs. Thus, engagement in the process of policy development is central to creating a health care system that meets the needs
of its constituents. Political activism and a commitment to policy development are central elements of professional nursing practice, and
the DNP graduate has the ability to assume a broad leadership role
on behalf of the public as well as the nursing profession (Ehrenreich,
2002). Health policy influences multiple care delivery issues, including health disparities, cultural sensitivity, ethics, the international-
ization of health care concerns, access to care, quality of care, health
care financing, and issues of equity and social justice in the delivery of
health care.

DNP graduates are prepared to design, influence, and implement
health care policies that frame health care financing, practice regulation,
access, safety, quality, and efficacy (IOM, 2001). Moreover, the DNP
graduate is able to design, implement, and advocate for health care policy that addresses issues of social justice and equity in health care. The
powerful practice experiences of the DNP graduate can become potent
influencers in policy formation. Additionally, the DNP graduate integrates these practice experiences with two additional skill sets: the ability to analyze the policy process and the ability to engage in politically
competent action (O'Grady, 2004).

The DNP graduate has the capacity to engage proactively in the development and implementation of health policy at all levels, including

institutional, local, state, regional, federal, and international levels. DNP graduates as leaders in the practice arena provide a critical interface between practice, research, and policy. Preparing graduates with the essential competencies to assume a leadership role in the development of health policy requires that students have opportunities to contrast the major contextual factors and policy triggers that influence health policy making at the various levels.

The DNP program prepares the graduate to:

1 Critically analyze health policy proposals, health policies, and related issues from the perspective of consumers, nursing, other health professions, and other stakeholders in policy and public forums.
2 Demonstrate leadership in the development and implementation of institutional, local, state, federal, and/or international health policy.
3 Influence policy makers through active participation on committees, boards, or task forces at the institutional, local, state, regional, national, and/or international levels to improve health care delivery and outcomes.
4 Educate others, including policy makers at all levels, regarding nursing, health policy, and patient care outcomes.
5 Advocate for the nursing profession within the policy and health care communities.
6 Develop, evaluate, and provide leadership for health care policy that shapes health care financing, regulation, and delivery.
7 Advocate for social justice, equity, and ethical policies within all health care arenas.

Essential VI: Interprofessional Collaboration for Improving Patient and Population Health Outcomes[1]

Today's complex, multitiered health care environment depends on the contributions of highly skilled and knowledgeable individuals from multiple professions. In order to accomplish the IOM mandate for safe, timely, effective, efficient, equitable, and patient-centered care in a complex environment, health care professionals must function as highly collaborative teams (AACN, 2004; IOM, 2003; O'Neil, 1998). DNP

---

[1] The use of the term *collaboration* is not meant to imply any legal or regulatory requirements or implications.

members of these teams have advanced preparation in the interprofessional dimension of health care that enable them to facilitate collaborative team functioning and overcome impediments to interprofessional practice. Because effective interprofessional teams function in a highly collaborative fashion and are fluid depending upon the patients' needs, leadership of high performance teams changes. Therefore, DNP graduates have preparation in methods of effective team leadership and are prepared to play a central role in establishing interprofessional teams, participating in the work of the team, and assuming leadership of the team when appropriate.

The DNP program prepares the graduate to:

1   Employ effective communication and collaborative skills in the development and implementation of practice models, peer review, practice guidelines, health policy, standards of care, and/or other scholarly products.
2   Lead interprofessional teams in the analysis of complex practice and organizational issues.
3   Employ consultative and leadership skills with intraprofessional and interprofessional teams to create change in health care and complex health care delivery systems.

Essential VII: Clinical Prevention and Population Health for Improving the Nation's Health

Clinical prevention is defined as health promotion and risk reduction/ illness prevention for individuals and families. *Population health* is defined to include aggregate, community, environmental/occupational, and cultural/socioeconomic dimensions of health. Aggregates are groups of individuals defined by a shared characteristic such as gender, diagnosis, or age. These framing definitions are endorsed by representatives of multiple disciplines including nursing (Allan et al., 2004).

The implementation of clinical prevention and population health activities is central to achieving the national goal of improving the health status of the population of the United States. Unhealthy lifestyle behaviors account for over 50% of preventable deaths in the United States, yet prevention interventions are underutilized in health care settings. In an effort to address this national goal, *Healthy People 2010* supported the transformation of clinical education by creating an objective to increase the proportion of schools of medicine, nursing, and other health professionals that have a basic curriculum that includes the core competencies in health promotion and disease prevention (Allan et al., 2004; USHHS, 2000). DNP graduates engage in leadership to integrate and institutionalize evidence-based clinical prevention and population health services for individuals, aggregates, and populations.

Consistent with these national calls for action and with the longstanding focus on health promotion and disease prevention in nursing curricula and roles, the DNP graduate has a foundation in clinical prevention and population health. This foundation will enable DNP graduates to analyze epidemiological, biostatistical, occupational, and environmental data in the development, implementation, and evaluation of clinical prevention and population health. Current concepts of public health, health promotion, evidence-based recommendations, determinants of health, environmental/occupational health, and cultural diversity and sensitivity guide the practice of DNP graduates. In addition, emerging knowledge regarding infectious diseases, emergency/disaster preparedness, and intervention frame DNP graduates' knowledge of clinical prevention and population health.

The DNP program prepares the graduate to:

1   Analyze epidemiological, biostatistical, environmental, and other appropriate scientific data related to individual, aggregate, and population health.
2   Synthesize concepts, including psychosocial dimensions and cultural diversity, related to clinical prevention and population health in developing, implementing, and evaluating interventions to address health promotion/disease prevention efforts, improve health status/access patterns, and/or address gaps in care of individuals, aggregates, or populations.
3   Evaluate care delivery models and/or strategies using concepts related to community, environmental, and occupational health, and cultural and socioeconomic dimensions of health.

Essential VIII: Advanced Nursing Practice

The increased knowledge and sophistication of health care has resulted in the growth of specialization in nursing in order to ensure competence in these highly complex areas of practice. The reality of the growth of specialization in nursing practice is that no individual can master all advanced roles and the requisite knowledge for enacting these roles. DNP programs provide preparation within distinct specialties that require expertise, advanced knowledge, and mastery in one area of nursing practice. A DNP graduate is prepared to practice in an area of specialization within the larger domain of nursing. Indeed, this distinctive specialization is a hallmark of the DNP.

Essential VIII specifies the foundational practice competencies that cut across specialties and are seen as requisite for DNP practice. All DNP graduates are expected to demonstrate refined assessment skills and base practice on the application of biophysical, psychosocial, behavioral, sociopolitical, cultural, economic, and nursing science as appropriate in their area of specialization.

DNP programs provide learning experiences that are based in a variety of patient care settings, such as hospitals, long-term care settings, home health, and/or community settings. These learning experiences should be integrated throughout the DNP program of study, to provide additional practice experiences beyond those acquired in a baccalaureate nursing program. These experiential opportunities should be sufficient to inform practice decisions and understand the patient care consequences of decisions. Because a variety of differentiated roles and positions may be held by the DNP graduate, role preparation for specialty nursing practice, including legal and regulatory issues, is part of every DNP program's curricula.

The DNP program prepares the graduate to:

1   Conduct a comprehensive and systematic assessment of health and illness parameters in complex situations, incorporating diverse and culturally sensitive approaches.
2   Design, implement, and evaluate therapeutic interventions based on nursing science and other sciences.
3   Develop and sustain therapeutic relationships and partnerships with patients (individual, family, or group) and other professionals to facilitate optimal care and patient outcomes.
4   Demonstrate advanced levels of clinical judgment, systems thinking, and accountability in designing, delivering, and evaluating evidence-based care to improve patient outcomes.
5   Guide, mentor, and support other nurses to achieve excellence in nursing practice.
6   Educate and guide individuals and groups through complex health and situational transitions.
7   Use conceptual and analytical skills in evaluating the links among practice, organizational, population, fiscal, and policy issues.

INCORPORATION OF SPECIALTY-FOCUSED COMPETENCIES INTO DNP CURRICULA

DNP education is by definition specialized, and DNP graduates assume a variety of differing roles upon graduation. Consequently, a major component of DNP curricula focuses on providing the requisite specialty knowledge for graduates to enact particular roles in the larger health care system. While all graduates demonstrate the competencies delineated in *DNP Essentials* I through VIII, further DNP preparation falls into two general categories: roles that specialize as an advanced practice nurse (APRN) with a focus on care of individuals, and roles that specialize in practice at an aggregate, systems, or organizational level. This distinction is important as APRNs face different licensure, regulatory, credentialing, liability, and reimbursement issues than those who practice at an aggregate, systems, or organizational level. As a result, the specialty content preparing DNP graduates for various practices will differ substantially.

It is noteworthy that specialties evolve over time, and new specialties may emerge. It is further recognized that APRN and aggregate/systems/organizational foci are not rigid demarcations. For example, the specialty of community health may have DNP graduates who practice in APRN roles providing direct care to individuals in communities; or community health DNP graduates may focus solely on programmatic development with roles fitting more clearly into the aggregate focus.

The specialized competencies, defined by the specialty organizations, are a required and major component of the DNP curriculum. Specialty organizations develop competency expectations that build upon and complement *DNP Essentials* I though VIII. ***All DNP graduates, prepared as APRNs, must be prepared to sit for national specialty APRN certification. However, all advanced nursing practice graduates of a DNP program should be prepared and eligible for national, advanced specialty certification, when available.***

Advanced Practice Nursing Focus

The DNP graduate prepared for an APRN role must demonstrate practice expertise, specialized knowledge, and expanded responsibility and accountability in the care and management of individuals and families. By virtue of this direct care focus, APRNs develop additional competencies in direct practice and in the guidance and coaching of individuals and families through developmental, health–illness, and situational transitions (Spross, 2005). The direct practice of APRNs is characterized by the use of a holistic perspective; the formation of therapeutic partnerships to facilitate informed decision making, positive lifestyle change, and appropriate self-care; advanced practice thinking, judgment, and skillful performance; and use of diverse, evidence-based interventions in health and illness management (Brown, 2005).

APRNs assess, manage, and evaluate patients at the most independent level of clinical nursing practice. They are expected to use advanced, highly refined assessment skills and employ a thorough understanding of pathophysiology and pharmacotherapeutics in making diagnostic and practice management decisions. **To ensure sufficient depth and focus, it is mandatory that a separate course be required for each of these three content areas: advanced health/physical assessment, advanced physiology/pathophysiology, and advanced pharmacology (see Appendix A).** In addition to direct care, DNP graduates emphasizing care of individuals should be able to use their understanding of the practice context to document practice trends, identify potential systemic changes, and make improvements in the care of their particular patient populations in the systems within which they practice.

Aggregate / Systems / Organizational Focus

DNP graduates in administrative, health care policy, informatics, and population-based specialties focus their practice on aggregates: populations, systems (including information systems), organizations, and state or national policies. These specialties generally do not have direct patient care responsibilities. However, DNP graduates practicing at the aggregate/systems/organization level are still called upon to define actual and emerging problems and design aggregate level health interventions. These activities require that DNP graduates be competent in advanced organizational, systems, or community assessment techniques, in combination with expert level understanding of nursing and related biological and behavioral sciences. The DNP graduate preparing for advanced specialty practice at the population/organizational/policy level demonstrates competencies in conducting comprehensive organizational, systems, and/or community assessments to identify aggregate health or system needs; working with diverse stakeholders for inter- or intra-organizational achievement of health-related organizational or public policy goals; and, designing patient-centered care delivery systems or policy level delivery models.

CURRICULAR ELEMENTS AND STRUCTURE

Program Length

Institutional, state, and various accrediting bodies often have policies that dictate minimum or maximum length and/or credit hours that accompany the awarding of specific academic degrees. Recognizing these constraints, it is recommended that programs designed for individuals who have already acquired the competencies in *The Essentials of Baccalaureate Education for Professional Nursing Practice* (AACN, 1998) be three calendar years, or 36 months of full-time study including summers, or four years on a traditional academic calendar.

Post-master's programs should be designed based on the DNP candidate's prior education, experience, and choice of specialization. Even though competencies for the DNP build and expand upon those attained through master's study, post-master's and post-baccalaureate students must achieve the same end-of-program competencies. Therefore, it is anticipated that a minimum of 12 months of full-time, post-master's study will be necessary to acquire the additional doctoral level competencies. The task force recommends that accrediting bodies should ensure that post-master's DNP programs have mechanisms in place to validate that students acquire all DNP end-of-program competencies. DNP programs, particularly post-master's options, should be efficient and manageable with regard to the number of credit hours required, and should avoid the development of unnecessarily long, duplicative, and/or protracted programs of study.

Practice Experiences in the Curriculum

DNP programs provide rich and varied opportunities for practice experiences aimed at helping graduates achieve the essential and specialty competencies upon completion of the program. In order to achieve the DNP competencies, programs should provide a minimum of 1,000 hours of practice post-baccalaureate as part of a supervised academic program. Practice experiences should be designed to help students achieve specific learning objectives related to the *DNP Essentials* and specialty competencies. These experiences should be designed to provide systematic opportunities for feedback and reflection. Experiences include in-depth work with experts from nursing as well as other disciplines and provide opportunities for meaningful student engagement within practice environments. Given the intense practice focus of DNP programs, practice experiences are designed to help students build and assimilate knowledge for advanced specialty practice at a high level of complexity. Therefore, end-of-program practice immersion experiences should be required to provide an opportunity for further synthesis and expansion of the learning developed to that point. These experiences also provide the context within which the final DNP product is completed.

Practice immersion experiences afford the opportunity to integrate and synthesize the essentials and specialty requirements necessary to demonstrate competency in an area of specialized nursing practice. Proficiency may be acquired through a variety of methods, such as attaining case requirements, patient or practice contact hours, completing specified procedures, demonstrating experiential competencies, or a combination of these elements. Many specialty groups already extensively define various minimal experiences and requirements.

Final DNP Project

Doctoral education, whether practice or research, is distinguished by the completion of a specific project that demonstrates synthesis of the student's work and lays the groundwork for future scholarship. For practice doctorates, requiring a dissertation or other original research is contrary to the intent of the DNP. The DNP primarily involves mastery of an advanced specialty within nursing practice. Therefore, other methods must be used to distinguish the achievement of that mastery. Unlike a dissertation, the work may take a number of forms. One example of the final DNP product might be a practice portfolio that includes the impact or outcomes due to practice and documents the final practice synthesis and scholarship. Another example of a final DNP product is a practice change initiative. This may be represented by a pilot study, a program evaluation, a quality improvement project, an evaluation of a new practice model, a consulting project, or an integrated critical literature review. Additional examples of a DNP final product could include manuscripts submitted for publication, systematic review, a research utilization project, practice topic dissemination, substantive involvement in a larger endeavor, or other practice project. The theme that links these forms of scholarly experiences is the use of evidence to improve either practice or patient outcomes.

The final DNP project produces a tangible and deliverable academic product that is derived from the practice immersion experience and is reviewed and evaluated by an academic committee. The final DNP product documents outcomes of the student's educational experiences, provides a measurable medium for evaluating the immersion experience, and summarizes the student's growth in knowledge and expertise. The final DNP product should be defined by the academic unit and utilize a form that best incorporates the requirements of the specialty and the institution that is awarding the degree. Whatever form the final DNP product takes, it will serve as a foundation for future scholarly practice.

DNP PROGRAMS IN THE ACADEMIC ENVIRONMENT: INDICATORS OF QUALITY IN DOCTOR OF NURSING PRACTICE PROGRAMS

Practice-focused doctorates are designed to prepare experts in nursing practice. The academic environments in which these programs operate must provide substantial access to nursing practice expertise and opportunities for students to work with and learn from a variety of practice experts including advanced clinicians, nurse executives, informaticists, or health policy makers. Thus, schools offering the DNP should have faculty members, practice resources, and an academic infrastructure that support a high-quality educational program and provide students with the opportunities to develop expertise in nursing practice. Similar to the need for PhD students to have access to strong research environments, DNP students must have access to strong practice environments, including faculty members who practice, environments characterized by continuous improvement, and a culture of inquiry and practice scholarship.

Faculty Characteristics

Faculty members teaching in DNP programs should represent diverse backgrounds and intellectual perspectives in the specialty areas for which their graduates are being prepared. Faculty expertise needed in these programs is broad and includes a mix of doctorally prepared research-focused and practice-focused faculty whose expertise will support the educational program required for the DNP. In addition to faculty members who are nurses, faculty members in a DNP program may be from other disciplines.

Initially, during the transition, some master's-prepared faculty members may teach content and provide practice supervision, particularly in early phases of post-baccalaureate DNP curriculum. Once a larger pool of DNP graduates becomes available, the faculty mix can be expected to shift toward predominately doctorally prepared faculty members.

The Faculty and Practice

Schools offering DNP programs should have a faculty cohort that is actively engaged in practice as an integral part of their faculty role. Active practice programs provide the same type of applied learning environment for DNP students as active research programs provide for PhD students. Faculty should develop and implement programs of scholarship that represent knowledge development from original research for some faculty and application of research in practice for others. Faculty, through their practice, provide a learning environment that exemplifies rapid translation of new knowledge into practice and evaluation of practice-based models of care.

Indicators of productive programs of practice scholarship include extramural grants in support of practice innovations; peer-reviewed publications and presentations; practice-oriented grant review activities; editorial review activities; state, regional, national, and international professional activities related to one's practice area; policy involvement; and development and dissemination of practice improvement products such as reports, guidelines, protocols, and tool kits.

Practice Resources and Clinical Environment Resources

Schools with DNP programs should develop, expand, sustain, and provide an infrastructure for extensive collaborative relationships with practice systems or sites and provide practice leadership in nursing and other fields. It is crucial for schools offering the DNP to provide or have access to practice environments that exemplify or aspire to the best in professional nursing practice, practice scholarship in nursing education, and provide opportunities for interprofessional collaboration (AACN, 2001a). Strong and explicit relationships need to exist with practice sites that support the practice and scholarship needs of DNP students, including access to relevant patient data and access to patient populations (e.g., direct access to individuals, families, groups, and communities) (AACN, 1999). Practice affiliations should be designed to benefit jointly the school and the practice sites. Faculty practice plans should also be in place that encourage and support faculty practice and scholarship as part of the faculty role.

Academic Infrastructure

The academic infrastructure is critical to the success of all DNP programs. Sufficient financial, personnel, space, equipment, and other resources should be available to accomplish attainment of DNP program goals and to promote practice and scholarship. Administrative as well as infrastructure support should reflect the unique needs of a practice-focused doctoral program. For example, this support would be evident in the information technology, library holdings, clinical laboratories and equipment, and space for academic and practice initiatives that are available for student learning experiences.

Academic environments must include a commitment to the practice mission. This commitment will be manifest through processes and structures that reflect a reconceptualization of the faculty role whereby teaching, practice, and practice-focused scholarship are integrated. This commitment is most apparent in systems that are consistent with Boyer's recommendations for broader conceptualization of scholarship and institutional reward systems for faculty scholarship (Boyer, 1990). Whether or not tenure is available for faculty with programs of scholarly practice, appropriate reward systems should be in place that endorse and validate the importance of practice-based faculty contributions. Formal faculty practice plans and faculty practice committees help institutionalize scholarly practice as a component of the faculty role and provide support for enhancing practice engagement. Faculty practice should be an essential and integrated component of the faculty role.

APPENDIX A

I. ADVANCED HEALTH/PHYSICAL ASSESSMENT

Advanced health/physical assessment includes the comprehensive history, physical and psychological assessment of signs and symptoms, pathophysiologic changes, and psychosocial variations of the patient (individual, family, or community). If the patient is an individual, the assessment should occur within the context of the family and community and should incorporate cultural and developmental variations and needs of the patient. The purpose of this comprehensive assessment is to develop a thorough understanding of the patient in order to determine appropriate and effective health care, including health promotion strategies.

There is a core of general assessment content that every advanced practice nurse must have. Specifics and additional assessment related to various specialties (e.g., women's health, mental health, anesthesiology, pediatrics) should be further addressed and refined in that specialty's course content within each program. Health/physical assessment must also be used as a base and be reinforced in all clinical experiences and practicum courses.

Individuals entering an advanced practice nursing program are expected to possess effective communication and patient teaching skills. Although these are basic to all professional nursing practice, preparation in the advanced practice nursing role must include continued refinement and strengthening of increasingly sophisticated communication and observational skills. Health/physical assessment content must rely heavily on the development of sensitive and skilled interviewing.

Course work should provide graduates with the knowledge and skills to:

1 Demonstrate sound critical thinking and clinical decision making;
2 Develop a comprehensive database, including complete functional assessment, health history, physical examination, and appropriate diagnostic testing;
3 Perform a risk assessment of the patient, including the assessment of lifestyle and other risk factors;
4 Identify signs and symptoms of common emotional illnesses;
5 Perform basic laboratory tests and interpret other laboratory and diagnostic data;
6 Relate assessment findings to underlying pathology or physiologic changes;
7 Establish a differential diagnosis based on the assessment data; and
8 Develop an effective and appropriate plan of care for the patient that takes into consideration life circumstance and cultural, ethnic, and developmental variations.

II. ADVANCED PHYSIOLOGY/PATHOPHYSIOLOGY

The advanced practice nurse should possess a well-grounded understanding of normal physiologic and pathologic mechanisms of disease, which serves as one primary component of the foundation for clinical assessment, decision making, and management. The graduate should be able to relate this knowledge "to interpreting changes in normal function that result in symptoms indicative of illness" and in assessing an individual's response to pharmacologic management of illnesses (NONPF, 1995, p. 152). Every student in an advanced practice nursing program should be taught a basic physiology/pathophysiology course. Additional physiology and pathophysiology content relevant to the specialty area may be taught in the specialty courses. In addition to the core course, content should be integrated throughout all clinical and practicum courses and experiences. The course work should provide the graduate with the knowledge and skills to:

1   Compare and contrast physiologic changes over the life span;
2   Analyze the relationship between normal physiology and pathological phenomena produced by altered states across the life span;
3   Synthesize and apply current research-based knowledge regarding pathological changes in selected disease states;
4   Describe the developmental physiology, normal etiology, pathogenesis, and clinical manifestations of commonly found/seen altered health states; and
5   Analyze physiologic responses to illness and treatment modalities.

III. ADVANCED PHARMACOLOGY

Every APRN graduate should have a well-grounded understanding of basic pharmacologic principles, which includes the cellular response level. This area of core content should include both pharmacotherapeutics and pharmacokinetics of broad categories of pharmacologic agents. Although taught in a separate or dedicated course, pharmacology content should also be integrated into the content of Advanced Health/Physical Assessment and Advanced Physiology and Pathophysiology courses. Additional application of this content should also be presented within the specialty course content and clinical experiences of the program in order to prepare the APRN to practice within a specialty scope of practice.

As described above, the purpose of this content is to provide the graduate with the knowledge and skills to assess, diagnose, and manage (including the prescription of pharmacologic agents) a patient's common health problems in a safe, high-quality, cost-effective manner. The course work should provide graduates with the knowledge and skills to:

1 Comprehend the pharmacotherapeutics of broad categories of drugs;
2 Analyze the relationship between pharmacologic agents and physiologic/pathologic responses;
3 Understand the pharmacokinetics and pharmacodynamics of broad categories of drugs;
4 Understand the motivations of patients in seeking prescriptions and the willingness to adhere to prescribed regimens; and
5 Safely and appropriately select pharmacologic agents for the management of patient health problems based on patient variations, the problem being managed, and cost effectiveness.

APPENDIX B

DNP ESSENTIALS TASK FORCE

Donna Hathaway, PhD
Chair Dean
College of Nursing
University of Tennessee Health Science Center

Janet Allan, PhD
Dean, School of Nursing
University of Maryland

Ann Hamric, PhD
Associate Professor, School of Nursing
University of Virginia

Judy Honig, EdD
Associate Dean, School of Nursing
Columbia University

Carol Howe, DNSc
Professor, School of Nursing
Oregon Health and Science University

Maureen Keefe, PhD
Dean, College of Nursing
University of Utah

Betty Lenz, PhD
Dean, College of Nursing
The Ohio State University

(Sr.) Mary Margaret Mooney, DNSc
Chair, Department of Nursing
North Dakota State University—Fargo

Julie Sebastian, PhD
Assistant Dean, College of Nursing
University of Kentucky

Heidi Taylor, PhD
Head, Division of Nursing
West Texas A&M University

Edward S. Thompson, PhD
Director, Anesthesia Nursing Program
University of Iowa

Polly Bednash, PhD (*Staff Liaison*)
Executive Director
AACN

Joan Stanley, PhD (*Staff Liaison*)
Senior Director, Education Policy
AACN

Kathy McGuinn, MSN (*Staff Liaison*)
Director, Special Projects
AACN

REFERENCES

Allan, J., Agar Barwick, T., Cashman, S., Cawley, J. F., Day, C., Douglass, C. W., et al. (2004). Clinical prevention and population health: Curriculum framework for health professions. *American Journal of Preventive Medicine, 27*(5), 471–476.

American Association of Colleges of Nursing. (1996). *The essentials of master's education for advanced practice nursing.* Washington, DC: Author.

American Association of Colleges of Nursing. (1998). *The essentials of baccalaureate education for professional nursing practice.* Washington, DC: Author.

American Association of Colleges of Nursing. (1999). *Essential clinical resources for nursing's academic mission.* Washington, DC: Author.

American Association of Colleges of Nursing. (2001a). *Hallmarks of scholarly clinical practice.* Washington, DC: Author.

American Association of Colleges of Nursing. (2001b). *Indicators of quality in research-focused doctoral programs in nursing* (AACN Position Statement). Washington, DC: Author.

American Association of Colleges of Nursing. (2004). *AACN position statement on the practice doctorate in nursing.* Washington, DC: Author.

Boyer, E. L. (1990). *Scholarship reconsidered: Priorities of the professoriate.* Princeton, NJ: Carnegie Foundation for the Advancement of Teaching.

Brown, S. J. (2005). Direct clinical practice. In A. B. Hamric, J. A. Spross, & C. M. Hanson (Eds.), *Advanced practice nursing: An integrative approach* (3rd ed.), (pp. 143–185). Philadelphia: Elsevier Saunders.

DePalma, J. A., & McGuire, D. B. (2005). Research. In A. B. Hamric, J. A. Spross, & C. Hanson (Eds.), *Advanced practice nursing: An integrative approach* (3rd ed.), (pp. 257–300). Philadelphia: Elsevier Saunders.

Diers, D. (1995). Clinical scholarship. *Journal of Professional Nursing, 11*(1), 24–30.

Donaldson, S., & Crowley, D. (1978). The discipline of nursing. *Nursing Outlook, 26*(2), 113–120.

Ehrenreich, B. (2002). The emergence of nursing as a political force. In D. Mason, D. Leavitt, & M. Chaffee (Eds.), *Policy & politics in nursing and health care* (4th ed.), (pp. xxxiii–xxxvii). St. Louis, MO: Saunders.

Fawcett, J. (2005). *Contemporary nursing knowledge: Analysis and evaluation of nursing models and theories* (2nd ed.). Philadelphia: Davis.

Gortner, S. (1980). Nursing science in transition. *Nursing Research, 29,* 180–183.

Institute of Medicine. (1999). *To err is human: Building a safer health system.* Washington, DC: National Academies Press.

Institute of Medicine. (2001). *Crossing the quality chasm: A new health system for the 21st century.* Washington, DC: National Academies Press.

Institute of Medicine. (2003). *Health professions education: A bridge to quality.* Washington, DC: National Academies Press.

National Research Council of the National Academies. (2005). *Advancing the nation's health needs: NIH research training programs.* Washington. DC: National Academies Press.

National Organization of Nurse Practitioner Faculties. (1995). *Advanced nursing practice: Curriculum guidelines and program standards for nurse practitioner education.* Washington, DC: Author.

O'Grady, E. (2004). Advanced practice nursing and health policy. In J. Stanley (Ed.), *Advanced practice nursing emphasizing common roles* (2nd ed.), (pp. 374–394). Philadelphia: Davis.

O'Neil, E. H., & the PEW Health Professions Commission. (1998). *Recreating health professional practice for a new century: The fourth report of the Pew Health Professions Commission.* San Francisco: Pew Health Professions Commission.

Palmer, I. S. (1986). The emergence of clinical scholarship as a professional imperative. *Journal of Professional Nursing, 2*(5), 318–325.

Porter-O'Grady, T. (2003). Nurses as knowledge workers. *Creative Nursing, 9*(2), 6–9.

Sigma Theta Tau International. (1999). *Clinical scholarship white paper.* Indianapolis, IN: Author.

Spross, J. A. (2005). Expert coaching and guidance. In A. B. Hamric, J. A. Spross, & C. M. Hanson (Eds.), *Advanced practice nursing: An integrative approach* (3rd ed), (pp. 187–223). Philadelphia: Saunders.

United States Department of Health and Human Services. (2000). *Healthy people 2010.* McLean, VA: International Medical Publishing.

Appendix B

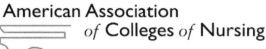

American Association *of* Colleges *of* Nursing

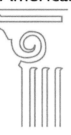

White Paper on the Education and Role of the Clinical Nurse Leader™

February 2007
(revised and approved by AACN Board
of Directors July 2007)

PREFACE

This document delineates *both* the entry-level competencies for all professional nurses (Essentials of Baccalaureate Education for Professional Nursing Practice 1998) and those competencies of the Clinical Nurse Leader™, an advanced generalist role. The competencies deemed necessary for the CNL role originally were delineated by the AACN Task Force on Education & Regulation II (TFERII) in the *Working Paper on the Clinical Nurse Leader* and accepted by the AACN Board (2003). Therefore, the competencies delineated here include all of the competencies deemed necessary for all graduates of a CNL education program.

In addition to the CNL graduate competencies, the Curriculum Framework, which includes required curricular components, required clinical experiences, and overarching end-of-program competencies, is included. These components provide the basis for the design and implementation of a master's or post-master's CNL education program and prepare the graduate to sit for the AACN CNL Certification Examination.

INTRODUCTION

Nursing education and the profession have an unparalleled opportunity and capability to address the critical issues that face the nation's current health care system. The American Association of Colleges of Nursing (AACN), representing baccalaureate and graduate schools of nursing, in collaboration with other health care organizations and disciplines, proposes a new Clinical Nurse Leader (CNL) role to address the ardent call for change being heard in today's health care system.

> *It is evident . . . that leadership in nursing . . . is of supreme importance at this time. Nursing has faced many critical situations in its long history, but probably none more critical than the situation it is now in, and none in which the possibilities, both of serious loss and of substantial advance, are greater. What the outcome will be depends in large measure on the kind of leadership the nursing profession can give in planning for the future and in solving stubborn and perplexing problems . . . if past experience is any criterion, little constructive action will be taken without intelligent and courageous leadership.*[1]

Isabel Maitland Stewart wrote those words over fifty years ago in her petition for education reform in nursing. Perhaps their most staggering revelation is that despite all of nursing's progress in recent decades, as a profession, nursing remains at the same 'critical' juncture where it was at the end of World War II. Despite the promise of university-based education for professional nursing, the health care system is in yet another nursing shortage with yet another call for 'intelligent and creative leadership.'

The *good* news is that nursing has the answers to the predominant health care dilemmas of the future, including the problems associated with normal human development, particularly aging; chronic illness management in all ages; health disparities associated with socioeconomic dislocations such as global migration, classism, sexism, and strategies for health promotion and disease prevention.

Each of these prevailing health problems is suited to the nursing paradigm. Their amelioration is what nursing students are educated to do. The advancement of medical science and technology has changed the landscape of health and illness. Not only are people living much longer, they are living with chronic illnesses that would have been fatal twenty years ago. This is true in adults and children, resulting in the need for providers who can manage the on-going health needs of persons of all ages. The necessity for practitioners who focus on the promotion of health and wellness and the prevention of disease has emerged as not only a good and wholesome thing to do in our society, but also as a means of addressing escalating medical costs. Whether working with older adults, children, refugees, ethnic minorities, persons with chronic illness, or whole communities, the predominant theme is the promotion and maintenance of health and the improvement of health care outcomes.

BACKGROUND

In November 1999, the Institute of Medicine (IOM) issued the comprehensive report on medical errors, *To Err is Human: Building a Safer Health System.* The report, extrapolating data from two previous studies, estimates that somewhere between 44,000 and 98,000 Americans die each year as a result of medical errors.[2] These numbers, even at the lower levels, exceed the number of people that die from motor vehicle accidents, breast cancer or AIDs. Total national costs of preventable adverse events (medical errors resulting in injury) were estimated to be between $17 billion and $29 billion, of which health care costs represented over one-half.[3] In addition, medication-related and other errors that do not result in actual harm are not only extremely costly as well but have a significant impact on the quality of care and health care outcomes. The IOM report also focused on the fragmented nature of the health care delivery system and the context in which health care is purchased as being major contributors to the high and inexcusable error rate.

In addition to the growing concern over health care outcomes, the United States is in the midst of a nursing shortage that is expected to intensify as baby boomers age and the need for health care grows. According to a study by Dr. Peter Buerhaus[4] and colleagues, published in the *Journal of the American Medical Association,* the U.S. will experience a 20% shortage in the number of nurses needed in our nation's health care system by the year 2020. This translates into a shortage of more than 400,000 RNs nationwide. The fall 2002 survey by the American Association of Colleges of Nursing (AACN) showed that enrollment in entry-level baccalaureate programs in nursing increased by 8% nationwide since fall 2001. This represents an increase of 5,316 enrollees and only 559 more graduates than the previous year. And despite these modest increases, enrollment is still down by almost 10% or 11,584 students from 1995.[5]

Several recent, landmark reports focus on the nursing shortage, the crisis in the health care system and proposed strategies for addressing these critical issues. The IOM report, *Crossing the Quality Chasm* (2001), stresses that the health care system as currently structured does not, as a whole, make the best use of its resources. The aging population and increased client demand for new services, technologies, and drugs contribute to the increase in health care expenditures, but also to the waste of resources. Recommendation two in the report calls on all health care organizations and professional groups to promote health care that is safe, effective, client-centered, timely, efficient, and equitable (p. 6).[6]

In a follow-up report, *Health Professions Education: A Bridge to Quality,* the Institute of Medicine[7] Committee on the Health Professions Education states, "All health professionals should be educated to deliver patient-centered care as members of an interdisciplinary team, emphasizing evidence-based practice, quality improvement approaches, and informatics (p. 3)."

The Joint Commission on Accreditation of Healthcare Organizations (JCAHO) in *Health Care at the Crossroads: Strategies for Addressing the Evolving Nursing Crisis*[8] urges that "the shortage of registered nurses has the potential to impact the very health and security of our society. . . . " Recommendations include proposals for transforming the workplace, aligning nursing education and clinical experience and providing financial incentives for health care organizations to invest in high quality nursing care.

The American Hospital Association (AHA) Commission on Workforce for Hospitals and Health Systems report, *In Our Hands: How Hospital Leaders Can Build a Thriving Workforce* (2002)[9], highlights the immediate and long-term critical workforce shortages facing hospitals. Five key recommendations include the need to foster meaningful work by designing health care to center on clients and the need to collaborate with professional associations and educational institutions to attract and prepare new health professions.

The Robert Wood Johnson Foundation in its commissioned 2002 report *Health Care's Human Crisis: The American Nursing Shortage*[10] takes a broad look at the underlying factors driving the nursing shortage. One of the key recommendations made is for the reinvention of nursing education and work environments to address and appeal to the needs and values of a new generation of nurses.

While there is ample evidence for the need to produce many more nurses to meet the pressing health care needs of society, this is not just a matter of increasing the volume of the nursing workforce. The nursing profession must produce quality graduates who:

- Are prepared for clinical leadership in all health care settings;
- Are prepared to implement outcomes-based practice and quality improvement strategies;
- Will remain in and contribute to the profession, practicing at their full scope of education and ability; and
- Will create and manage microsystems of care that will be responsive to the health care needs of individuals and families.[11,12]

In addition, unless nursing is able to create a professional role that will attract the highest quality women and men into nursing, we will not be able to fulfill our covenant with the public. The Clinical Nurse Leader (CNL) addresses the call for change.

The realities of a global society, expanding technologies, and an increasingly diverse population require nurses to master complex information, to coordinate a variety of care experiences, to use technology for health care delivery and evaluation of nursing outcomes, and to assist clients with managing an increasingly complex system of care. The extraordinary explosion of knowledge in all fields also requires an increased emphasis on lifelong learning. Nursing education must keep pace with these changes and prepare individuals to meet these challenges. Change, however, cannot occur in isolation. Nursing education must collaborate and work in tandem with the health care delivery system to design and test models for education and practice that are truly client-centered, generate quality outcomes, and are cost-effective. Significant changes must occur in both education and the practice setting to produce the delivery system desired by all constituents. New ways of educating health professionals, including inter-professional education and practice, and new practice models must be developed that better use available resources and address the health care needs of a rapidly growing, diverse population.

EDUCATING THE CLINICAL NURSE LEADER

In response to client care needs and to the health care delivery environment, the American Association of Colleges of Nursing (AACN) proposes the Clinical Nurse Leader (CNL) role. The design of this role has been done in collaboration with constituents from a broad array of expertise and leadership roles within the health care system. Participants at the Stakeholders' Reaction Panel Meeting (2003) confirmed that this role has emerged and is being further developed on an ad hoc basis. Individuals to fill this role are being recruited opportunistically based on available clinicians with appropriate experience, personal characteristics, and self-selection. Stakeholders affirmed the need to produce these clinicians through a formal degree-granting program of education.

The CNL is a leader in the health care delivery system across all settings in which health care is delivered, not just the acute care setting. The implementation of the CNL role, however, will vary across settings. The CNL role is not one of administration or management. The CNL functions within a microsystem and assumes accountability for health care outcomes for a specific group of clients within a unit or setting through the assimilation and application of research-based information to design, implement, and evaluate client plans of care. The CNL is a provider and a manager of care at the point of care to individuals and cohorts. The

CNL designs, implements, and evaluates client care by coordinating, delegating and supervising the care provided by the health care team, including licensed nurses, technicians, and other health professionals.

Ten Assumptions For Preparing Clinical Nurse Leaders

Assumption 1: Practice Is At The Microsystems Level

In addition to being direct care providers, the CNL is accountable for the care outcomes of clinical populations or a specified group of clients in a health care system. As clinical decision maker and care manager, the CNL coordinates the direct care activities of other nursing staff and health professionals. The CNL provides lateral integration of care services within a microsystem of care to effect quality client care outcomes. To prepare students for the CNL role, there must be a deliberate and integrated inclusion of leadership education and socialization that begins on the first day of the first class and continues throughout the CNL education program. For example, leadership content should be incorporated in every client care plan prepared by students so that each plan includes not only *clinical* actions for meeting the needs of the client but also an *organizational* plan for delegation of care to assisting personnel, registered nurses, and other health professionals, including the teaching and evaluation activities that would need to accompany such delegation. One leadership course taken in the last year of the CNL course of study is not sufficient to prepare the student who can perform as a beginning CNL upon graduation. Practice at the unit and systems level will require a shift in thinking on the part of faculty, with greater attention to context and the development of leadership skills throughout the curriculum. Students, as well, may have to be convinced that systems-level intervention, such as the implementation of best practices and the revision of guidelines and protocols for the management of clinical populations, is essential for professional practice and has a greater probability of generating superior and far-reaching outcomes.

Assumption 2: Client Care Outcomes Are The Measure Of Quality Practice

The performance of the CNL will be measured by the extent to which he or she succeeds in improving clinical and cost outcomes in individuals and groups of clients within a unit or setting, e.g. diminishing recidivism in schizophrenic clients; elimination of pressure ulcers in nursing home residents; reducing hospital length of stays for clients admitted with pneumonia; increasing participation in prenatal care and classes in a community. Professional nursing education must provide opportunities for students to isolate and describe clinical populations, e.g. adults with chronic obstructive pulmonary disease (COPD), well school-aged children or an urban neighborhood, and identify the clinical and cost outcomes that will improve safety, effectiveness, timeliness, efficiency, quality, and the degree to which they are client-centered. In the process, CNL students must learn how to compare desired outcomes with national and state standards and with those of other institutions. CNL education can make a significant contribution to the health of the public by emphasizing *common clinical conditions* that comprise the bulk of health care activity and cost and where professional nursing is likely to have the greatest impact on the health care system and outcomes. For example, in the past, nursing education has been dogged about assuring that every student has the opportunity to attend a birth but has never insisted that every student have the opportunity to manage a death, even though the vast majority of nurses are more likely to practice with clients who are at the end of life. Similarly, gerontology has not been a universal curriculum requirement even though persons over 65 use the lion's share of health resources nationally.

Assumption 3: Practice Guidelines Are Based On Evidence

The preparation of the CNL must include an unrelenting demand for evidence for every aspect of practice. While most higher education programs in nursing have made the transition from ritualistic, process-based teaching to an evidence-based, outcome orientation, many graduates do not routinely read professional journals and incorporate new evidence into practice. These leadership activities require skill in knowledge acquisition, working in groups, management of change, and dissemination of new knowledge to other health care professionals. Most professional nursing education programs have included a course in nursing research but often have neglected the more meaningful pursuit of clinical scholarship, i.e., the application of research to the clinical setting, the resolution of clinical problems, and dissemination of results.

In addition to justifying clinical actions based on evidence, the CNL student should have the opportunity, within his or her course of study, to seek and apply evidence that challenges current policies and procedures in a practice environment and to incorporate evidence into practice situations, including the education of other health care team members. Practical experience in the dissemination of clinical knowledge such as grand rounds, case presentations and journal clubs should be intrinsic to CNL education to ensure that the implementation of new evidence becomes embedded in practice.

Assumption 4: Client-Centered Practice Is Intra- And Interdisciplinary

For care to be client-centered, the providers who comprise the health care team must discuss the client's problem and agree on a common course of action. As the health care team member who has the most comprehensive knowledge of the client, the CNL necessarily will be responsible for coordinating the variety of team members participating in the plan of care. Currently, many students complete their course of study in nursing without having had the opportunity to work closely with physicians, physical therapists, social workers, pharmacists and others who are caring for the same client. Likewise, communication with other nurses who provide care to the same client(s) in other settings is seldom stressed. This lack of communication results in discontinuous and frequently unsafe, uncoordinated, inappropriate care. Learning to advocate for clients by communicating effectively with other interdisciplinary team members, including nurses in other settings, must start in CNL education programs with real experiences. Faculty members must role model this behavior and create opportunities for students to work with the other professions as well as with nursing staff. The opportunity to learn and work in an interdisciplinary venue teaches students how to be effective client care advocates and coordinators.

Assumption 5: Information Will Maximize Self-Care And Client Decision Making

Client participation traditionally has been a nursing goal; however, the stunning advances in science and technology—specifically informatics and genetics—have taken it to a new level. As participants in their own care, clients require in-depth, up-to-date knowledge about themselves, their specific health problems, and their treatment options. Health literacy is the foundation of independence, health promotion and disease prevention, all of which are hallmarks of excellence in nursing practice. CNL education requires comprehensive content in clinical genetics and clinical practice opportunities in genetics counseling, e.g. assisting clients to construct genealogies and identify family patterns of health problems. Clinical practica also must include educating clients and families—not just on how to perform a procedure at home but also the nature of the problem, and how they can acquire additional knowledge about the condition and support from others with similar problems. Teaching other direct care providers how to assist clients, families and communities to be health literate and independent managers of their own care is a system responsibility of the CNL that requires practice opportunities in the education program. In CNL education, a health literacy plan should be a component of each care plan and include family members and other care providers.

Assumption 6: Nursing Assessment Is The Basis For Theory And Knowledge Development

With the explosion of knowledge, the CNL or any other health professional can not know everything that is required for a safe, high quality clinical practice. The use of information technology for decision support for all clinicians will be critical and depends on the routine collection of data that documents the characteristics, conditions and outcomes for various clinical groups or populations. Assessment has been a core activity of nursing practice. To engage clients in therapeutic partnerships, the CNL must communicate with them and must first assess the individual, his or her health problems, and the context in which those problems are manifested in order to effectively communicate. In the future, assessment data not only will guide individual plans of care, but also will be classified (using a standardized language), stored, retrieved, analyzed and then integrated into information systems to continuously update decision support, and complete the cycle of evidence-based practice. CNL education must include an understanding of information systems and standardized languages, and how they relate to the improvement of clinical outcomes, continuous performance measures and decision support technology.

Assumption 7: Good Fiscal Stewardship Is A Condition Of Quality Care

Requesting more and more resources to support an essentially dysfunctional system is injudicious. However, attempting to drive costs down by withholding and rationing services is equally misguided. Accountability for the cost-effective and efficient use of human, environmental and material resources will rest with the CNL. This expectation requires an understanding of how to identify waste and manage resources within systems. For example, using a CNL to perform client care tasks that can be done as effectively by less prepared nursing personnel is poor fiscal stewardship; however, delegating certain activities to less prepared nursing personnel resulting in poorer client outcomes is also not fiscally sound management. The CNL student must understand the fiscal context in which he or she is practicing and how to identify the high cost/high volume activities, including how much procedures cost and how those costs compare nationally and across institutions. Managing the care of a clinical population or group can be compared to running a small business. The CNL needs to understand economies of scale, how to read a balance sheet, the difference between fixed and incremental costs, how to establish per unit costs, and some basic marketing strategies. Basic business skills and organizational theory must become accepted components of CNL education.

Assumption 8: Social Justice Is An Essential Nursing Value

Altruism, accountability, human dignity, integrity and social justice are the guiding values of the nursing profession. For the CNL, however, the value of social justice is particularly significant because it directly addresses disparities in health and health care. As one of only two goals of the Healthy People 2010 agenda, the elimination of health disparities requires an in-depth understanding of the impact of unequal distribution of wealth and a pluralistic health care system. As the health professional charged with the management of clinical unit or setting-based populations, the CNL will assume responsibility for addressing variations in clinical outcomes among various groups, including those most vulnerable. Although professional nursing education programs have included cultural competence and health disparities content in the curricula, such content seldom addresses the more comprehensive issue of social justice. The opportunity to work with clinical populations and even whole communities to assess and implement strategies that address health disparities is imperative in the education of the CNL and serves as a prelude to influencing policy formulation at the systems level.

Assumption 9: Communication Technology Will Facilitate The Continuity And Comprehensiveness Of Care

While the face-to-face clinic visit, home visit and hospital stay have been the traditional venues for provider-client interaction, technological advances in communication have made it possible for more sustained and ongoing contact with clients, families, and other caregivers. Four fifteen-minute visits per year in a physician's office are an insufficient and costly way to manage chronic illness, often resulting in untimely and inappropriate use of the most expensive health care services. The ability to develop and sustain therapeutic relationships, monitor the course of illness and health events on a continuous basis and provide care using varied and distance technologies is a necessary component of CNL education. Students must have the opportunity to diagnose, educate, treat and evaluate the care of clients, using distance and varied technology. Communication courses will include the range of interactions from face-to-face to electronic interactions with individuals and groups, as well as with the media, policy makers and public.

Assumption 10: The CNL Must Assume Guardianship For The Nursing Profession

The ability of professional nursing to fulfill its covenant with society and protect and promote the health of citizens and communities will depend on the health care leadership of the CNL. The CNL, with additional education, will be expected to assume positions in professional, policy and regulatory organizations/agencies, leadership positions in health care facilities, practice plans, and as faculty in institutions of higher education. The assumption of the CNL's leadership in the health care system, however, begins with entry into the education program and includes a clear expectation of the more advanced generalist's clinical practice role, including delegation to other licensed nurses. This socialization and leadership role preparation may be the most difficult dimension of CNL education and requires extensive socialization and actual practice, as well as modeling by faculty members and staff nurses. Leadership development activities must become a core component of the CNL curriculum and awarded credit accordingly.

THE ROLE OF THE CLINICAL NURSE LEADER

The CNL is a leader in the health care delivery system, not just the acute care setting but in all settings in which health care is delivered. The implementation of the CNL role, however, will vary across settings. The CNL role is not one of administration or management. The CNL assumes accountability for client care outcomes through the assimilation and application of research-based information to design, implement, and evaluate client plans of care. The CNL is a provider and manager of care at the point of care to individuals and cohorts of clients within a unit or health care setting. The CNL designs, implements, and evaluates client care by coordinating, delegating and supervising the care provided by the health care team, including licensed nurses, technicians, and other health professionals.

Fundamental aspects of the CNL role include:

- Leadership in the care of the sick in and across all environments;
- Design and provision of health promotion and risk reduction services for diverse populations;
- Provision of evidence-based practice;
- Population-appropriate health care to individuals, clinical groups/ units, and communities;
- Clinical decision-making;
- Design and implementation of plans of care;
- Risk anticipation;
- Participation in identification and collection of care outcomes;
- Accountability for evaluation and improvement of point-of-care outcomes;
- Mass customization of care;
- Client and community advocacy;
- Education and information management;

- Delegation and oversight of care delivery and outcomes;
- Team management and collaboration with other health professional team members;
- Development and leveraging of human, environmental and material resources;
- Management and use of client-care and information technology; and
- Lateral integration of care for a specified group of patients.

The CNL provides and manages care at the point of care to individuals, clinical populations and communities. In this role, the CNL is responsible for the clinical management of comprehensive client care, for individuals and clinical populations, along the continuum of care and in multiple settings, including virtual settings. The CNL is responsible for planning a client's contact with the health care system. The CNL also is responsible for the coordination and planning of team activities and functions. In order to impact care, the CNL has the knowledge and authority to **delegate** tasks to other health care personnel, as well as **supervise and evaluate** these personnel and the outcomes of care. Along with the authority, autonomy and initiative to design and implement care, the CNL is accountable for improving individual care outcomes and care processes in a quality, cost-effective manner.

As the use of technology expands and care is delivered not only across multiple settings but in virtual settings as well, the CNL has the knowledge and skills to deliver and coordinate care across settings using up-to-date technology.

Risk anticipation, the ability to critically evaluate and anticipate risks to client safety, is a critical component of the CNL role. At the systems level (risk to any client) and the individual level (account for client history, co-morbidities, etc.) it is necessary to anticipate risk when new technology, equipment, treatment regimens or medication therapies are introduced. Tools for risk analysis, e.g. failure mode evaluation analysis, root cause analysis, and quality improvement methodologies, and the potential use of large data sets, are important concepts in the armamentarium of the CNL.

Mass customization, the ability to profile patterns of need and tailor interventions, is a key component of the CNL role. The CNL uses an evidence-based approach by identifying patterns, and modifying interventions to meet specific needs of individuals, clinical populations, or communities within a microsystem. This approach to health care requires the CNL to collaborate with individuals in providing client-focused care.

Client and community advocacy is a hallmark of the CNL role. As a client advocate the CNL assumes accountability for the delivery of high quality care, including the evaluation of care outcomes and provision of leadership in improving care. Historically, the nursing role has emphasized partnership with clients—whether individuals, families, groups, or communities—in order to foster and support active participation in determining health care decisions. In addition, the CNL advocates for improvement in the institution or health care system and the nursing profession.

In this role, the CNL also assumes the role of *educator,* preparing individuals, families, or cohorts of clients for self-care and a maximal level of functioning and wellness. The CNL serves as an information manager, with state-of-the art knowledge regarding research findings and health information resources. As advocates and educators with state-of-the-art knowledge, the CNL helps clients acquire, interpret, and use information related to health care, illness, and health promotion. Health information available to clients is often overwhelming or confusing; the CNL serves as an information manager, assisting clients in accessing, understanding, evaluating and applying health-related information. To maximize wellness, health promotion, and risk reduction, the CNL designs and implements education programs for cohorts of clients, with particular emphasis on those with chronic illnesses. In addition, the CNL provides education and guidance to other health professionals to whom care is delegated.

The CNL is responsible for the provision and management of care in and across all environments. The CNL focuses not only on individual-level health care, but also manages, monitors, and manipulates the environment to foster health. In addition, the CNL develops, leverages, and serves as a *steward of the environment and human and material resources* while coordinating client care. The CNL role requires knowledge and skill in biotechnology and information technology as these relate to direct nursing care, health education, and the management and coordination of care.

The CNL is a *member and leader of health care teams* that deliver treatment and services in an evolving health care system. The CNL brings a unique blend of knowledge, judgment, skills, and caring to the health care team. As a leader and partner with other members of the health care team, the CNL seeks collaboration and consultation with other health professionals as necessary in the design, coordination and evaluation of client care outcomes.

As a health care provider and leader who functions autonomously and as a member of an interdisciplinary health care team, the CNL is responsible for his/her own professional identity and practice. Self-awareness and self-evaluation are utilized to enhance professional relationships, improve communication and improve quality of care outcomes.

The role of the CNL requires strong critical thinking, communication and assessment skills, and the demonstration of a balance of intelligence, confidence, understanding, and compassion. Membership in any profession, and more specifically as a CNL, requires the development and acquisition of an appropriate set of values and an ethical framework. As advocates for high quality care for all individuals, the CNL is knowledgeable and active in the political and regulatory processes defining health care delivery and systems of care.

A defining feature of the CNL role is a strong focus on health promotion, risk reduction and population-based health care. As advances in science and technology allow us to predict future health problems, the CNL will be called upon to design and implement measures to modify risk factors and promote engagement in healthy lifestyles. While the CNL will continue to provide and coordinate care to the sick, many will engage in direct interaction with groups and communities for the purpose of health promotion, secondary prevention, and risk reduction.

The CNL is committed to lifelong learning and willing to assume responsibility for planning one's professional career. As a professional committed to lifelong learning, the CNL is able to define his or her professional self by purposeful and structured educational experiences for the ongoing improvement of practice competence and improved practice outcomes.

In summary, the role of the beginning CNL encompasses the following broad areas:

- **Clinician:** designer/coordinator/integrator/evaluator of care to individuals, families, groups, communities, and populations; able to understand the rationale for care and competently deliver this care to an increasingly complex and diverse population in multiple environments. The CNL provides care at the point of care to individuals across the lifespan with particular emphasis on health promotion and risk reduction services.

- ■ *Outcomes manager:* synthesizes data, information and knowledge to evaluate and achieve optimal client outcomes.
- ■ *Client advocate:* adept at ensuring that clients, families and communities are well-informed and included in care planning and is an informed leader for improving care. The CNL also serves as an advocate for the profession and the interdisciplinary health care team.
- ■ *Educator:* uses appropriate teaching principles and strategies as well as current information, materials and technologies to teach clients, groups and other health care professionals under their supervision.
- ■ *Information manager:* able to use information systems and technology that put knowledge at the point of care to improve health care outcomes;
- ■ *Systems analyst/Risk anticipator:* able to participate in systems review to improve quality of client care delivery and at the individual level to critically evaluate and anticipate risks to client safety with the aim of preventing medical error.
- ■ *Team Manager:* able to properly delegate and manage the nursing team resources (human and fiscal) and serve as a leader and partner in the interdisciplinary health care team.
- ■ *Member of a profession:* accountable for the ongoing acquisition of knowledge and skills to effect change in health care practice and outcomes and in the profession.
- ■ *Lifelong Learner:* recognizes the need for and actively pursues new knowledge and skills as one's role and needs of the health care system evolves.

EDUCATION FOR THE CLINICAL NURSE LEADER ROLE

To prepare individuals for this multi-faceted role, several components are essential. These components are liberal education, professional values, core competencies, core knowledge, and role development.

Liberal Education

Liberal education is the critical foundation for and an integral component of the clinical nurse leader's education. Liberal learning provides a solid basis for the development of clinical judgment skills. While providing a framework of knowledge in the arts and sciences, liberal education also promotes critical thinking, the basis for clinical judgment and ethical decision making. Through liberal education, students encounter a diversity of thought that enables them to integrate varied perspectives and divergent experiences. Knowledge from the arts and sciences enables the professional person to develop and use personal standards, to make reasoned choices when evidence is scant or conflicting, and to articulate ideas effectively in written and spoken forms. Well-grounded liberal education helps ensure that clinical nurse leaders practice within a context of broad-based knowledge.

Liberal education is not a separate or distinct segment of professional education, but an integrated educational experience, recognized and valued as an ongoing, lifelong process. Courses in the arts, sciences, and humanities provide a forum for the study of values, ethical principles, and the physical world, as well as opportunities to reflect and apply knowledge to professional practice.

Many colleges and universities have adopted a liberal education core. This core provides an effective base of knowledge and cognitive skills for the educated person. CNL students who participate in joint learning activities with students from other disciplines derive significant benefits from such exposure and contribute to the learning of students from other disciplines.

While specific courses and curricula will vary, CNL education must include a strong base in the physical and social sciences as well as learning experiences in philosophy, the arts, and humanities. Recent and evolving trends in health care require particular emphasis on learning related to: economics, environmental science, epidemiology, genetics, gerontology, global perspectives, informatics, organizations and systems, and communications.

The successful integration of liberal education and professional education requires guidance from faculty to help students build bridges between general concepts and practice. Making these connections enables students to use what they have learned to understand situations in nursing practice. Students must be accountable for previous knowledge just as faculty are responsible for building on that foundation, facilitating cognitive skill development, and encouraging lifelong learning. Professional education must build upon the competencies, knowledge and skills acquired through liberal education courses.

Liberal education provides the CNL with the ability to:

- develop and use higher-order problem-solving and critical thinking skills;
- integrate concepts from behavioral, biological, and natural sciences in order to understand self and others;
- interpret and use quantitative data;
- use the scientific process and scientific data as a basis for developing, implementing, and evaluating nursing interventions;
- apply knowledge regarding social, political, economic, environmental and historical issues to the analysis of societal, professional and client problems;
- synthesize information and knowledge as a key component of critical thinking and decision making;
- communicate effectively in a variety of written and spoken formats;
- engage in effective working relationships;
- appreciate cultural differences and bridge cultural and linguistic barriers;
- understand the nature of human values;
- develop and articulate personal standards against which to measure new ideas and experiences; and
- appreciate and understand the character of professions.

Professional Values

Education for the CNL role should facilitate the development of professional values and value-based behaviors. Values are beliefs or ideals to which an individual is committed and which are reflected in patterns of behavior. Professional values are the foundation for practice; they guide interactions with clients, colleagues, other professionals, and the public. Values provide the framework for commitment to client welfare, fundamental to professional nursing practice and critical decision-making processes.

The values and sample professional behaviors listed below epitomize the CNL. The CNL, guided by these values, demonstrates ethical behaviors in the provision of safe, humanistic health care. The sample behaviors are not mutually exclusive and may result from more than one value. Conversely, the value labels provided are intended to encapsulate a core set of values and behaviors that can be elaborated in a variety of ways.

Altruism is a concern for the welfare and well-being of others. In professional practice, altruism is reflected by the CNL's concern for the welfare of clients, other nurses, and other health care providers. Sample professional behaviors include:

- demonstrates understanding of cultures, beliefs, and perspectives of others;
- advocates for clients, particularly the most vulnerable;
- takes risks on behalf of clients and colleagues; and
- mentors other professionals.

Accountability is the right, power, and competence to act. Accountability includes the autonomy, authority and control of one's actions and decisions. Professional practice reflects accountability when the CNL evaluates individual and group health care outcomes and modifies treatment or intervention strategies to improve outcomes. The CNL also uses risk analysis tools and quality improvement methodologies at the systems level to anticipate risk to any client and intervenes to decrease the risk. Sample professional behaviors include:

- evaluates client care and implements changes in care practices to improve outcomes of care;
- serves as a responsible steward of the environment, and human and material resources while coordinating care;
- uses an evidence-based approach to meet specific needs of individuals, clinical populations or communities;
- manages, monitors and manipulates the environment to foster health and health care quality; and
- prevents or limits unsafe or unethical care practices.

Human Dignity is respect for the inherent worth and uniqueness of individuals and populations. In professional practice, human dignity is reflected when the CNL values and respects all clients and colleagues. Sample professional behaviors include:

- provides culturally competent and sensitive care;
- protects the client's privacy;
- preserves the confidentiality of clients and health care providers; and
- designs care with sensitivity to individual client needs.

Integrity is acting in accordance with an appropriate code of ethics and accepted standards of practice. Integrity is reflected in professional practice when the CNL is honest and provides care based on an ethical framework that is accepted within the profession. Sample professional behaviors include:

- provides honest information to clients and the public;
- documents care accurately and honestly;
- seeks to remedy errors made by self or others; and
- demonstrates accountability for own actions and those of other health care team members under the supervision of the CNL.

Social Justice is upholding moral, legal, and humanistic principles. This value is reflected in professional practice when the CNL works to assure equal treatment under the law and equal access to quality health care. Sample professional behaviors include:

- supports fairness and non-discrimination in the delivery of care;
- promotes universal access to health care; and
- encourages legislation and policy consistent with the advancement of nursing care and health care.

Educational efforts and the process of socialization into the profession must build upon, and as appropriate, modify values and behavior patterns developed early in life. Values are difficult to teach as part of professional education. Nevertheless, faculty must design learning opportunities that support empathic, sensitive, and compassionate care for individuals, groups, and communities; that promote and reward honesty and accountability; that make students aware of social and ethical issues; and that nurture students' awareness of their own value systems, as well as those of others.

Core Competencies

Core competencies listed will be acquired over the course of a student's academic program from a simple application to a more complex level of integration. These core competencies should be assessed across this continuum from entry to graduation. Each of the competencies defined can be attributed, at some level or degree, to a wide range of roles and health care providers. The CNL through graduate education attains a level of competence to provide high quality, client-focused, accountable practice as a health care professional and clinical leader.

Critical Thinking

Critical thinking underlies independent and interdependent decision making. Critical thinking includes questioning, analysis, synthesis, interpretation, inference, inductive and deductive reasoning, intuition, application, and creativity. Critical thinking includes the ability to use evidence gathered through personal experiences and through the research of others in evaluating and designing models and plans of care.

Course work or clinical experiences should provide the graduate with the knowledge and skills to:

- use nursing and other appropriate theories and models, and an appropriate ethical framework;
- apply research-based knowledge from nursing and the sciences as the foundation for evidence-based practice;
- use clinical judgment and decision-making skills to:
  - bring multiple perspectives into the interpretation of situations and problems encountered;
  - evaluate evidence and relevant arguments appropriately, including assumptions that influence behavior;
  - communicate the results of thinking clearly and in context.
- engage in self reflection and collegial dialogue about professional practice;
- evaluate nursing care outcomes through the acquisition of data and the questioning of inconsistencies, allowing for the revision of actions and goals;
- engage in creative problem solving; and
- design and redesign client care based on analysis of outcomes and evidence-based knowledge.

Communication

Communication is a complex, ongoing, interactive process and forms the basis for building interpersonal relationships. Communication includes critical listening, critical reading, and quantitative literacy, as well as oral, nonverbal, and written communication skills. Communication requires the effective use of a wide range of media, including not only face-to-face interactions, but also rapidly evolving technological modalities. Further, communication includes effectiveness in group interactions, particularly in task-oriented, convergent, and divergent group situations. Communication requires the acquisition of skills necessary to interact and collaborate with other members of the interdisciplinary health care team as well as to develop a therapeutic alliance with the client.

Course work or clinical experiences should provide the graduate with the knowledge and skills to:

- demonstrate communication skills during assessment, intervention, evaluation, and teaching;
- express oneself effectively using a variety of media in a variety of contexts;
- help clients access and interpret the meaning and validity of health information available through multiple and varied sources and formats;
- establish and maintain effective working relationships within an interdisciplinary team;
- communicate confidently and effectively with other health care workers both in collegial and subordinate positions;
- adapt communication methods to clients with special needs, e.g., sensory or psychological disabilities;
- produce clear, accurate, and relevant writing;
- develop a therapeutic alliance and relationship with the client;
- use therapeutic communication within the nurse-client relationship;
- appropriately, accurately, and effectively communicate with diverse groups and disciplines using a variety of strategies;
- access and use data and information from a wide range of resources;
- provide relevant and sensitive health education information and counseling to clients;
- thoroughly and accurately document interventions and nursing outcomes;
- elicit and clarify client preferences and values; and
- manage group processes to meet care objectives and complete health care team responsibilities.

Assessment

Assessment skills form the foundation of evidence-based practice. Assessment includes gathering information about the health status of the client, analyzing and synthesizing those data, making judgments about nursing interventions based on the findings, evaluating and managing individual care outcomes. Assessment also includes understanding the family, community, or population and using data from organizations and systems in planning and delivering care. The analysis of systems and outcomes data sets to anticipate individual client risk and improve quality of care delivery is another critical form of assessment.

Course work or clinical experiences should provide the graduate with the knowledge and skills to:

- perform a risk assessment of the individual, including lifestyle, family and genetic history, and other risk factors;
- perform a holistic assessment of the individual across the life span, including a health history which includes spiritual, social, cultural, and psychological assessment, as well as a comprehensive physical exam;
- assess physical, cognitive, and social functional ability of the individual in all developmental stages, with particular attention to changes due to aging;
- assess an individual's level of pain or discomfort;
- evaluate an individual's capacity to assume responsibility for self care;
- perform a health assessment of the family;
- perform a community health risk assessment for diverse populations;
- perform an assessment of the environment in which health care is provided;
- use assessment findings to diagnose, plan, deliver, and evaluate quality care; and,
- use risk analysis tools to anticipate risks to client safety.

Nursing Technology And Resource Management

Acquisition and use of client care technology and nursing procedures are required for the delivery of nursing care. While the CNL must understand the principles related to and be adept at performing skills, major roles will include teaching, delegating, and supervising the performance of skilled tasks by others and behaviors of others. Consequently, graduates must approach their understanding and use of skills in a sophisticated theoretical and analytic manner. The application of nursing science and client care technology is necessary to perform nursing procedures. The acquisition of new skills is an ongoing component of health care and nursing care delivery and will depend on the practice setting, specialty area of practice, and the development of new knowledge and technologies. Skill development should focus on the mastery of core scientific principles that underlie all skills, thus preparing the graduate to incorporate current and future technologies into the evaluation and delivery of client care.

The teaching, learning, and assessment of any given skill should serve as an exemplar that focuses as much on helping the student learn the process for lifelong self-mastery of needed skills, as on the learning of the specific skill itself. The emphasis must be on helping students identify those skills essential for nursing practice and understanding the scientific principles that underlie the application of these skills.

The CNL should be able to perform, teach, delegate, and supervise nursing procedures with safety and competence. As nursing practice changes to meet the needs of contemporary health care delivery, required skills and expectations related to the graduate's competence must be reviewed and revised.

Course work or clinical experiences should provide the graduate with the knowledge and skills to:

- provide effective health teaching to clients, using appropriate materials, technologies, resources, and formats;
- evaluate effectiveness of health teaching by self and others;
- delegate safely client care activities, determine client staffing ratios, and evaluate the outcomes of such actions;
- evaluate the environmental impact on health care outcomes;
- evaluate the appropriate use of products in the delivery of health care;
- evaluate and manage the efficient use of human and material resources; and,
- design, coordinate, and evaluate plans of care.

Health Promotion, Risk Reduction, And Disease Prevention

The CNL must have a strong theoretical foundation in health promotion, illness prevention and maintenance of the client's (individual, family, group or community) function in health and illness. Health promotion and disease prevention is an integral part of nursing practice.

Health promotion requires knowledge about health risks and methods to prevent or reduce these risks in individuals and populations. Knowledge of the expected growth and development of individuals across the life span is essential. Disease prevention knowledge includes methods to keep an illness or injury from occurring, diagnosing and treating a disease early in its course, and preventing further deterioration of an individual's functioning due to disease. Health promotion and disease prevention enable individuals to achieve and maintain an optimal level of wellness across the life span, and decrease disparities in health that exist across populations. Effective health promotion, risk reduction, and disease prevention also require effective teaching and evaluation skills and knowledge, including knowledge and use of available resources, teaching and communication methods, and learning principles.

Course work or clinical experiences should provide the graduate with the knowledge and skills to:

- assess protective and predictive factors that influence the health of clients;
- assess genetic factors and risks that influence the health of individuals;
- foster strategies for health promotion, risk reduction, and disease prevention across the life span;
- develop clinical and health promotion programs for individuals and groups to reduce risk, prevent disease, and prevent disease sequelae, particularly related to chronic illness;
- recognize the need for and implement risk reduction strategies to address social and public health issues, including mass casualty incidents, environmental exposures, societal and domestic violence, family abuse, sexual abuse, and substance use;
- use information technologies to communicate health promotion and disease prevention information to the client in a variety of settings;
- develop an awareness of complementary modalities and their usefulness in promoting health;
- help clients and populations access and interpret health information to identify healthy lifestyle behaviors;
- initiate community partnerships to establish health promotion goals and implement strategies to meet those goals;
- evaluate the efficacy of health promotion and education modalities for use in a variety of settings and with diverse populations;

- demonstrate sensitivity to personal and cultural definitions of health;
- use epidemiological, social, and environmental data to draw inferences regarding the health status of client populations;
- develop and monitor comprehensive, holistic plans of care that address the health promotion and disease prevention needs of client populations;
- incorporate theories and research in generating teaching and counseling strategies to promote and preserve health and healthy lifestyles in client populations;
- foster a multidisciplinary approach to discuss strategies and garner multifaceted resources to empower client populations in attaining and maintaining maximal functional wellness; and
- influence regulatory, legislative, and public policy in private and public arenas to promote and preserve health communities.

Illness And Disease Management

Illness and disease management requires knowledge about pharmacology, pathophysiology of disease, and assessment and management of symptoms across the life span with particular emphasis on the chronicity and sequelae of illness. Also, knowledge about the social, physical, psychological, and spiritual responses of the individual and family or caregiver to disease and illness is required. The goal is to maximize the quality of life and maintain optimal level of functioning throughout the course of illness, including end of life. The CNL uses case management skills and principles to provide and supervise continuous care within specific episodes and across episodes of illness and disease.

The CNL also uses knowledge of illness and disease management to provide research-based care to populations, perform risk assessment, and design plans of care.

Course work or clinical experiences should provide the graduate with the knowledge and skills to:

- assess and manage physical and psychological symptoms related to disease and treatment;
- assess, design, and provide interventions for the moderation of pain and suffering;
- administer pharmacological and non-pharmacological therapies;

- demonstrate sensitivity to personal and cultural influences on individual and family reactions to the illness experience and end of life;
- maintain, restore, and optimize an individual's level of functioning;
- anticipate and manage complications of disease progression;
- assist clients to achieve a peaceful end of life;
- anticipate, plan for, and manage physical, psychological, social, and spiritual needs of the client and family or caregiver;
- use case management skills and principles in the delivery and supervision of client care across a continuum;
- apply principles of infection control;
- evaluate and anticipate risks to client safety using risk analysis tools;
- synthesize data, information and knowledge on client outcomes and modify interventions to improve health care outcomes; and
- identify, report, and appropriately respond to a mass casualty incident.

Information And Health Care Technologies

Information technology includes traditional and developing methods of discovering, retrieving, and using information in nursing practice. Knowledge of and effective use of information technology is necessary for evidence-based practice and for effective, appropriate health teaching. The use of technology is critical for the documentation and evaluation of client care outcomes.

Health care technology includes methods and equipment designed to provide assessment data and support anatomic and physiological function. The CNL applies technology in the delivery of client care and intercedes between the client and technology; therefore, the ability to assess the need for, as well as the efficacy and use of, technology is critical.

Course work or clinical experiences should provide the graduate with the knowledge and skills to:

- use information and communication technologies to document and evaluate client care, advance client education, and enhance the accessibility of care;
- use appropriate technologies in the process of assessing and monitoring clients;

- work in an interdisciplinary team to make ethical decisions regarding the application of technologies and the acquisition of data;
- adapt the use of technologies to meet client needs;
- teach clients about health care technologies;
- protect the safety and privacy of clients in relation to the use of health care and information technologies;
- use information technologies to enhance one's own knowledge base;
- access, critique, and analyze information sources; and
- disseminate health care information appropriately using a variety of means.

Ethics

Ethics includes values, codes, and principles that govern decisions in nursing practice, conduct, and relationships. Skill and knowledge in resolving conflicts related to role obligations and personal beliefs are necessary. The CNL is able to identify potential and actual ethical issues arising from practice and help clients and other health care providers address such issues; therefore, knowledge of ethics and ethical decision making is critical. The CNL serves as a client advocate within the health care delivery and policy systems. In addition, the CNL interfaces between the client and the health care delivery system to protect the rights of clients and to effect quality outcomes.

Course work or clinical experiences should provide the graduate with the knowledge and skills to:

- clarify personal and professional values and recognize their impact on decision making and professional behavior;
- apply a professional nursing code of ethics and professional guidelines to clinical practice;
- apply an ethical decision-making framework to clinical situations that incorporates moral concepts, professional ethics, and law and respects diverse values and beliefs;
- apply legal and ethical guidelines to advocate for client well-being and preferences;
- apply communication, negotiation, and mediation skills to the ethical decision-making process;
- demonstrate accountability for one's own practice;
- take action to prevent or limit unsafe or unethical health and nursing care practices by others;

- enable individuals and families to make quality-of-life and end-of-life decisions and achieve a peaceful death;
- assume responsibility for lifelong learning and accountability for current practice and health care information and skills;
- identify and analyze common ethical dilemmas and the ways in which these dilemmas impact client care;
- evaluate ethical methods of decision making and engage in an ethical decision-making process;
- evaluate ethical decision making from both a personal and organizational perspective and develop an understanding of how these two perspectives may create conflicts of interest;
- identify areas in which a personal conflict of interest may arise and propose resolutions or actions to resolve the conflict;
- understand the purpose of an ethics committee's role in health care delivery systems; and,
- assume accountability for the quality of one's own practice and client care outcomes related to nursing care.

Human Diversity

Human diversity includes understanding the ways cultural, ethnic, socioeconomic, linguistic, religious, and lifestyle variations are expressed. The CNL is able to apply knowledge of the effects these variations have on health status and response to health care. The CNL is well prepared to care for the aging population and to help all individuals and families make decisions about life-extending technologies and treatments within the context of their values, as well as physical, emotional, and spiritual health parameters.

Skills in a second language are highly desirable for the CNL. Opportunities should be provided for students to learn languages and to integrate language skills into clinical practice.

Course work or clinical experiences should provide the graduate with the knowledge and skills to:

- understand how human behavior is affected by culture, ethnicity, language, religion, gender, lifestyle and age;
- provide holistic care that addresses the needs of diverse populations across the life span;
- work collaboratively with health care providers from diverse backgrounds;

- understand the effects of health and social policies on persons from diverse backgrounds, particularly vulnerable populations;
- advocate for health care that is sensitive to the needs of clients, with particular emphasis on the needs of vulnerable populations;
- perform a community assessment, using appropriate epidemiological principles;
- differentiate and compare the wide range of cultural norms and health care practices of diverse groups;
- define, design, and implement culturally competent health care;
- ensure that systems meet the needs of the population(s) served and are culturally relevant;
- recognize the variants in health, including physiological variations, in a wide range of cultural, ethnic, age, and gender groups that may influence the assessment and plan of care; and
- practice in collaboration with a multicultural workforce.

Global Health Care

Global health care knowledge includes an understanding of the implications of living with transportation and information technology that link all parts of the world. Information about the effects of the global community on such areas as disease transmission, health policy, and health care economics is required. Global health care also includes an understanding of and ability to share information with health care providers across disciplines, cultures, and geographic boundaries.

Course work or clinical experiences should provide the graduate with the knowledge and skills to:

- understand the global environment in which health care is provided;
- adapt or seek consultation to adapt client care in response to global environmental factors (e.g., international law, international public health, geopolitics, and geo-economics);
- access and communicate health care information with health care providers from other disciplines, cultures and countries;
- understand the effect of the global community on intentional and non-intentional disease transmission;
- understand the effect of the global community on health policy and health care economics; and
- define or identify the global dimensions of health care.

Health Care Systems And Policy

Knowledge of health care systems includes an understanding of the organization and environment in which nursing and health care is provided. Health care policy shapes health care systems and helps determine accessibility, accountability, and affordability. The CNL has an understanding of the economies of care, a beginning understanding of business principles, and an understanding of how to work within and affect change in systems.

In an environment with ongoing changes in the organization and financing of health care, it is imperative that all CNL graduates have a keen understanding of health care policy, organization, and financing of health care. The purpose of this content is to prepare a graduate to provide quality cost-effective care, to participate in the implementation of care in a variety of health care systems, and to assume a leadership role in the managing of human, fiscal, and physical health care resources at the microsystem level.

Course work or clinical experiences should provide the graduate with the knowledge and skills to:

- use systems theory in the design, delivery, and evaluation of health care;
- understand how health care delivery systems are organized and financed, and the effect on client care;
- understand basic business and economic principles and practices, including budgeting, product testing, marketing, and organizational models;
- manage a budget at the client care level;
- use quality improvement methods in evaluating individual and aggregate client care and for self-improvement;
- identify the economic, legal, and political factors that influence health care delivery;
- participate in political processes and grass roots legislative efforts to influence health care policy on behalf of clients or the profession;
- differentiate and delineate legislative and regulatory processes;
- articulate the interaction between regulatory controls and quality control within the health care delivery system;
- evaluate local, state and national socioeconomic and health policy issues and trends;

- articulate health care issues and concerns to elected and appointed officials, both public and private, and to health care consumers;
- interpret health care research for consumers and officials;
- serve as a consumer advocate on health issues;
- articulate the significance of the CNL and other nursing roles to policymakers, health care providers, and consumers.
- incorporate knowledge of cost factors in delivering care; and
- understand the effect of legal and regulatory processes on nursing practice and health care delivery.

Provider And Manager Of Care

The CNL uses theory and research-based knowledge in the design, co-ordination, and evaluation of the delivery of client care. The CNL is a leader in the interdisciplinary health care team in the planning, delivery, and evaluation of client-focused care.

Course work or clinical experiences should provide the graduate with the knowledge and skills to:

- integrate theory and research-based knowledge from the arts, humanities, and sciences to develop a foundation for practice;
- apply appropriate knowledge of major health problems and cultural diversity in performing nursing interventions;
- demonstrate knowledge of the importance and meaning of health and illness for the client in providing nursing care;
- apply health care technologies to maximize optimal outcomes for clients;
- participate in research that focuses on the efficacy and effectiveness of nursing interventions;
- delegate, supervise, and evaluate the performance of nursing interventions;
- incorporate principles of quality management into the plan of care;
- use outcome measures to evaluate effectiveness of care;
- perform direct and indirect therapeutic interventions;
- develop a comprehensive plan of care in collaboration with the client;
- serve as the client's advocate;
- prepare the client for a maximal level of self-care;
- integrate care with other members of the interdisciplinary health care team; and

- evaluate and assess the usefulness of integrating traditional and complementary health care practices.

Designer/Manager/Coordinator Of Care

The CNL takes primary responsibility for the design, coordination, and management of health care across the life span and in all types of health care settings. The CNL provides and coordinates comprehensive care for clients: individuals, families, groups, and communities, in multiple and varied settings. Using information from numerous sources, the CNL guides the client through the health care system. Skills essential to this role development are communication, collaboration, negotiation, delegation, coordination, and evaluation of interdisciplinary work, and the application, design and evaluation of outcome-based practice models.

Course work or clinical experiences should provide the graduate with the knowledge and skills to:

- assume a horizontal leadership role in the health care team;
- coordinate and manage care to meet the special needs of vulnerable populations, including the frail elderly, in order to maximize independence and quality of life;
- coordinate the health care of individuals across the life span using principles and knowledge of interdisciplinary models of care delivery and case management;
- coordinate the health care of clients across settings;
- delegate, supervise and evaluate the nursing care given by others while retaining accountability for the quality of care given to the client;
- organize, manage, and evaluate the development of strategies to promote healthy communities;
- organize, manage, and evaluate the functioning of a team or unit;
- use appropriate evaluation methods to analyze the quality of nursing care;
- use cost-benefit analysis and variance data in providing and evaluating care;
- intervene or modify nursing care, based on risk anticipation analysis and other evidence-based information to improve health care outcomes; and
- promote interdisciplinary cohesion through the use of task-oriented, convergent and divergent group process skills.

Member Of A Profession

The CNL has an understanding of the role and responsibilities of a professional and leader in the health care delivery system, as well as knowledge and experiences that encourage the embracing of lifelong learning, the incorporation of professionalism into practice, and identification with the values of the profession. The CNL is responsible for the professional presentation of self. In addition, a critical component of the CNL role is the development and mentoring of the next generation of professionals.

Course work or clinical experiences should provide the graduate with the knowledge and skills to:

- understand the history, philosophy and responsibilities of the nursing profession;
- incorporate professional nursing standards and accountability into practice;
- assume responsibility for the professional presentation of oneself;
- establish oneself as a credible health care provider and resource;
- advocate for professional standards of practice using organizational and political processes;
- understand limits to one's scope of practice and adhere to licensure law and regulations;
- articulate to the public the values of the profession as they relate to client welfare;
- negotiate and advocate for the role of the professional nurse as a member of the interdisciplinary health care team;
- develop personal goals for professional development and continuing education;
- participate in professional organizations, working to support agendas that enhance both high quality, cost-effective health care, and the advancement of the profession; and
- support and mentor individuals entering into and training for professional nursing practice.

TRANSITION TO THE PRACTICE SETTING

An extended clinical experience, prior to graduation, mentored by an experienced Clinical Nurse Leader, is critical to the effective implementation of the role. As the CNL role evolves, through established academic-practice partnerships, those who initially mentor the CNL students and new graduates will have emerged as CNLs as a result of their expertise and continued learning. The intensive immersion into the role and practice expectations during this experience reflect the health care delivery system and provide the student with the opportunity to practice in a chosen health care environment(s) and to integrate knowledge and skills acquired throughout the education experience. The integrative experience must occur in an evolved practice environment that allows for the full implementation of this new role. In addition, a strong interdisciplinary practice focus must be embedded into the experience.

Finally, a comprehensive assessment of the knowledge and skills assimilated throughout the educational experience serves as the culmination of the CNL education. At the end of the transition stage, measurable outcomes will demonstrate the student's:

- ability to integrate knowledge and skills acquired throughout the didactic and clinical education experiences,
- understanding of one's accountability for practice outcomes, and
- ability to practice interdependently and independently beyond the novice stage.

Significant impact on the health care system and successful outcomes will not be realized unless there is true partnership and collaboration between the education and practice arenas. Individuals educated in the new CNL role cannot go into health care settings that have not also evolved. Successful change in both the practice environment and nursing education requires committed and active partnerships between education and practice in nursing and with other health professions. Improvement in health care outcomes, the ultimate goal, can only occur through meaningful and dedicated partnerships and a willingness to commit significant resources and energy to realizing this goal.

NOTES

1 Stewart, I. M. (1953). *The Education of Nurses*. New York: The Macmillan Company.
2 Institute of Medicine. (2000). *To Err Is Human: Building a Safer Health System*. Washington, DC: National Academy Press, p. 1.
3 Johnson, W. G., Brennan, T. A., Newhouse, J. P., Leape, L. L., Lawthers, A. G., Hiatt, H. H., & Weiler, P. C. (1992). The

economic consequences of medical injuries. *Journal of the American Medical Association, 267,* 2487–2492.

4   Buerhaus, P., Staiger, D. O., & Auerbach, D. I. (2000, June 12). Implications of an Aging Registered Nurse Workforce. *Journal of the American Medical Association, 283,* 22.

5   Berlin, L. E., Stennett J, & Bednash, G. D. (2003). *2002–2003 Enrollment and Graduations in Baccalaureate and Graduate Programs in Nursing.* Washington, DC: American Association of Colleges of Nursing.

6   Institute of Medicine. (2001). *Crossing the Quality Chasm.* Washington, DC: The National Academies Press.

7   Institute of Medicine. (2003). *Health Professions Education: A Bridge to Quality.* Washington, DC: The National Academies Press.

8   Joint Commission on Accreditation of Healthcare Organizations. (2002). *Health Care at the Crossroads, Strategies for Addressing the Evolving Nursing Crisis.* Chicago: Author.

9   American Hospital Association Commission on Workforce for Hospitals and Health Systems. (2002). *In Our Hands, How Hospital Leaders Can Build a Thriving Workforce.* Chicago: American Hospital Association.

10   Kimball, B. & O'Neill, E. (2002). *Health Care's Human Crisis: The American Nursing Shortage.* Princeton, NJ: The Robert Wood Johnson Foundation.

11   Batalden, P. B., Nelson, E. C., Edwards, W. H., Godfrey, M. M., & Mohr, J. J. (2003, November). Microsystems in Health care. Part 9. Developing Small Clinical Units to attain Peak Performance. *Joint Commission Journal on Quality and Safety,* 29(11), 575–585.

12   Mohr, J. J., Barach, P., Cravero, J. P., Blike, G. T., Godfrey, M. M., Batalden, P. B., & Nelson, E. C. (2003, August). Microsystems in Health Care: Part 6. Designing Patient Safety into the Microsystem. *Joint Commission Journal on Quality and Safety,* 29(8), 401–408.

AACN Task Force On Education And Regulation II

Chairperson

Jean Bartels, PhD, RN
Chair, School of Nursing

Georgia Southern University
Statesboro, Georgia

Members

Carol Allen, PhD, RN
Chair, Department of Nursing
Oakwood College
Huntsville, Alabama

Lauren Arnold, PhD, RN
Senior Director and Operations Analyst
Tenet Health
Dallas, Texas

Tina DeLapp, EdD, RN
Director, School of Nursing
University of Alaska—Anchorage
Anchorage, Alaska

Melanie Dreher, PhD, RN, FAAN
Dean, College of Nursing
University of Iowa
Iowa City, Iowa

Donna Hartweg, PhD, RN
Director, School of Nursing
Illinois Wesleyan University
Bloomington, Illinois

Elizabeth Lenz, PhD, RN, FAAN
Dean, College of Nursing
The Ohio State University
Columbus, Ohio

Terry Miller, PhD, RN
Dean, School of Nursing
Pacific Lutheran University
Tacoma, Washington

Roberta Olson, PhD, RN
Dean, College of Nursing
South Dakota State University
Brookings, South Dakota

Cathy Rick, RN, CNAA, CHE
Chief Nursing Officer
Department of Veterans Affairs
Washington, District of Columbia

Elias Vasquez, PhD, NNP, PNP, FAAN
Assistant Professor, School of Nursing
Department of Child, Women's and Family Health,
University of Maryland
Baltimore, Maryland

AACN Staff

Polly Bednash, PhD, RN, FAAN
Executive Director

Joan Stanley, PhD, RN, CRNP
Director of Education Policy

Reaction Panel

Lauren Arnold, PhD, RN
Senior Director and Operations Analyst
Tenet Health
Dallas, Texas

Jean Bartels, PhD, RN (*TF Chair*)
Director, School of Nursing
Georgia Southern University
Statesboro, Georgia

Geraldine Bednash, PhD, RN, FAAN
Executive Director
American Association of Colleges of Nursing
Washington, District of Columbia

Karen N. Drenkard, RN, MSN, CNAA
Chief Nurse Executive
Inova Health System
Falls Church, Virginia

Donna Dorsey, MS, RN
President
National Council of State Boards of Nursing
Chicago, Illinois

Catherine J. Futch, MN, RN, CNAA
President-Elect
American Academy of Ambulatory Care Nursing
Pitman, New Jersey

Tim Henderson, MSPH
National Conference of State Legislatures
Primary Care Resource Center
Washington, District of Columbia

Jean Johnson, PhD, RNC, FAAN
Senior Associate Dean, Health Sciences
George Washington University
Washington, District of Columbia

Marian Osterweis, PhD
Executive Vice President and Director
Division of Global Health
Association of Academic Health Centers
Washington, District of Columbia

Joy F. Reed, EdD, RN
President
Association of State and Territorial Directors of Nursing
Raleigh, North Carolina

Cathy Rick, RN, CNAA, CHE
Chief Nursing Officer
Department of Veterans Affairs
Washington, District of

Mary Smolenski, EdD, RN, CS, FNP
Director of Certification Services
American Nurses Credentialing Center
Washington, District of Columbia

Joan Stanley, PhD, RN, CRNP
Director of Education Policy
American Association of Colleges of Nursing
Washington, District of Columbia

Jolene Tornabeni, RN, MA, FACHE, FAAN
Executive Vice President and Chief
Operating Officer
Inova Health System
Falls Church, Virginia

Michael Whitcomb, MD
Senior Vice President for Medical Education
Association of American Medical Colleges
Washington, District of Columbia

Consultant

Maureen K. Robinson
Bethesda, Maryland

ADDENDUM: CLINICAL NURSE LEADER CURRICULUM FRAMEWORK

Assumptions Regarding CNL Curriculum/Education

1 The CNL education program culminates in a master's degree in nursing.
2 The CNL graduate will be prepared as a generalist.
3 The CNL graduate will be competent to provide care at the point of care.
4 The CNL graduate will be prepared in clinical leadership for setting specific practice throughout the health care delivery system.
5 The CNL graduate is eligible to matriculate to a practice- or research-focused doctoral program.
6 The CNL graduate is prepared with advanced nursing knowledge and skills but does not meet the criteria for Advanced Practice Nursing (APRN) scope of practice.

Expectations Of CNL Curriculum/Education

1 All programs, including those designed for post high school entry or second-degree programs (Model C), build upon the competencies in the *Essentials of Baccalaureate Education for Professional Nursing Practice* (AACN, 1998).
2 All students graduating from a CNL program will have a strong liberal education background in the arts and sciences.
3 CNL graduates will have content at the undergraduate or graduate level in the following areas:
   - Anatomy and physiology
   - Microbiology
   - Epidemiology
   - Statistics

- Health Care Policy
4 All CNL graduates will have additional *graduate-level* content that builds upon an undergraduate foundation in:

- Health assessment
- Pharmacology
- Pathophysiology

Although not required, it is recommended that the CNL curriculum include three separate graduate-level courses in these three content areas. Having clinical nursing leaders at the point of care with a strong background in these three areas is seen as imperative from the practice perspective. In addition, the inclusion of these three separate courses facilitates the transition of these master's program graduates into the DNP specialty programs.

5 All programs will demonstrate achievement of the five IOM health professions core competencies: quality improvement, interdisciplinary team care, patient-centered care, evidence-based practice and utilization of informatics.

6 All education programs, working with their practice partners, will designate a clinical mentor/preceptor for each CNL student.

7 To prepare a CNL graduate with the necessary graduate-level content **post attainment of the baccalaureate competencies,** it is recommended that the graduate-level curriculum, including the clinical immersion experience, be designed within a 12–15 month, 3 semesters or 4 quarters time frame, depending upon the institution's academic calendar. The rationale for this recommendation is that this is an advanced generalist model; preparation is not required to develop the specialist focus of an advanced practice nurse.

GRADUATE-LEVEL CURRICULAR ELEMENTS OF THE CNL CURRICULUM

The presentation of these curricular elements assumes previous attainment of the competencies delineated in the AACN *Essentials of Baccalaureate Education for Professional Nursing Practice* (1998).

The CNL education program at the graduate level builds upon the direct-care nursing skills acquired in an undergraduate baccalaureate nursing program or in the initial pre-licensure component of the CNL education program. Building upon these direct care skills, the CNL graduate-level curriculum develops a solid foundation in policy/organization, outcomes management, nursing leadership and care management.

The Curriculum Framework is intended to serve as a guide when developing the graduate CNL curriculum. **The bolded and numbered headings identified in the diagram below are required components of the curriculum.** Ten major curricular threads are integrated throughout the curriculum; therefore, **each course in the curriculum should address each of the identified threads.** The remaining bulleted items or specific content areas under each numbered heading in the diagram are recommendations and are included to assist you in the development of the curriculum.

CNL CURRICULUM FRAMEWORK FOR CLIENT-CENTERED HEALTH CARE

<u>**Nursing Leadership**</u>
  I. Horizontal Leadership
 II. Effective Use of Self
III. Advocacy
 IV. Conceptual Analysis of the CNL Role
  V. Lateral Integration of Care

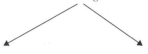

<u>**Clinical Outcomes Management**</u> ◄───────► <u>**Care Environment Management**</u>

  I. Illness/Disease Management
- Care management
- Client outcomes
- Builds on and expands the baccalaureate foundation in:
  1. Pharmacology
  2. Physiology/pathophysiology
  3. Health Assessment

 II. Knowledge Management
- Epidemiology
- Biostatistics
- Measurement of client outcomes

III. Health Promotion and Disease Reduction/Prevention Management
- Risk assessment
- Health literacy
- Health education and counseling

 IV. Evidence-Based Practice
- Clinical decision making
- Critical thinking
- Problem identification
- Outcome measurement

  I. Team Coordination
- Delegation
- Supervision
- Interdisciplinary care
- Group process
- Handling difficult people
- Conflict resolution

 II. Health Care Finance/Economics
- Medicare and Medicaid/Reimbursement
- Resource allocation
- Health care technologies
- Health care finance & socioeconomic principles

III. Health Care Systems & Organizations
- Unit level health care delivery/Microsystems of care
- Complexity theory
- Managing change theories

 IV. Health Care Policy
  V. Quality Management/Risk Reduction/Patient Safety
 VI. Informatics

Major Threads Integrated Throughout Curriculum
    I. Critical thinking/Clinical decision making
   II. Communication
  III. Ethics
   IV. Human diversity/cultural competence
    V. Global Health Care
   VI. Professional development in the CNL role
  VII. Accountability
 VIII. Assessment
   IX. Nursing technology and resource management
    X. Professional values, including social justice

Clinical Experiences In the CNL Education Program

The total number of clinical hours should be determined by the CNL program faculty. However, the CNL program must meet the following requirements:

- Each CNL student completes a total of 400–500 clinical contact hours as part of the formal education program.
- A minimum of 300–400 of these hours will be in an immersion experience in practice in the CNL role with a designated clinical preceptor **and** a faculty partner over a 10–15 week period of time.
- The immersion experience will include weekly opportunities with other CNL students, faculty and mentors to dialogue on issues and assess experiences, particularly the implementation of the role.
- The immersion experience is in addition to the clinical experiences integrated throughout the education program.

CNL Certification™

After successful completion of the formal CNL education program, including the 10–15 week immersion experience, the CNL graduate will be eligible to sit for the CNL Certification Examination™ developed under the auspices of the American Association of Colleges of Nursing.

Post-Graduation Mentorship

After graduation, it also is strongly recommended that a clinical mentor be designated by the health care institution for each newly employed CNL graduate. The length of the mentorship will depend upon the length of previous experiences and demonstration of successful attainment of the CNL competencies and practice in the CNL role. The nursing mentor should be educated at the graduate level and have the necessary expertise and understanding of the CNL role and practice expectations.

END-OF-PROGRAM COMPETENCIES & REQUIRED CLINICAL EXPERIENCES FOR THE CLINICAL NURSE LEADER

This section delineates the competencies expected of every graduate of a CNL master's degree education program. A minimum set of clinical experiences required to attain the end-of-program competencies also is included.

GRADUATE LEVEL CURRICULUM ELEMENTS	CNL ROLE FUNCTIONS	CNL ROLE EXPECTATIONS	END-OF-PROGRAM COMPETENCIES	REQUIRED CLINICAL EXPERIENCES
	Advocate	■ Keeps clients well informed ■ Includes clients in care planning ■ Advocates for the profession ■ Works with interdisciplinary team ■ Strives to achieve social justice within the microsystem	Effects change through advocacy for the profession, interdisciplinary health care team and the client. Communicates effectively to achieve quality client outcomes and lateral integration of care for a cohort of clients.	Identify clinical and cost outcomes that improve safety, effectiveness, timeliness, efficiency, quality and client-centered care. Communicate within a conflict milieu with nurses and other health care professionals who provide care to the same clients in that setting and in other settings. Review and evaluate patient care guidelines/ protocols and implement a guideline to address an identified patient care issue like pain management or readiness for discharge; follow-up to evaluate the impact on the issue. Discover, disseminate and apply evidence for practice and for changing practice. Participate in development of or change in policy within the health care organization. Identify potential equity and justice issues within the health care setting related to client care.
	Nursing Leadership			

Nursing Leadership		
Advocate		Present to appointed/elected officials regarding a health care issue with a proposal for change.
		Analyze the care of a patient cohort and the care environment in light of ANA Nursing Standards of Care and the Code of Ethics.
		Analyze interdisciplinary patterns of communication and chain of command both internal and external to the unit that impact care.
Member of a Profession	■ Effects change in health care practice ■ Effects change in health outcomes ■ Effects change in the profession	Actively pursues new knowledge and skills as the CNL role, needs of clients, and the health care system evolve.
		Develop a lifelong learning plan for self.
		Speak at a public engagement to a public forum.
		Participate in a professional organization/or agency wide committee.
Team Manager	■ Properly delegates and manages ■ Uses team resources effectively ■ Serves as leader/ partner on interdisciplinary team	Properly delegates and utilizes the nursing team resources (human and fiscal) and serves as a leader and partner in the interdisciplinary health care team.
		Design, coordinate, & evaluate plans of care for a cohort of patients incorporating patient/family input and team member input.
		Monitor/delegate care in the patient care setting.
		Present to the multidisciplinary team a cost saving idea that improves patient care outcomes and improves efficiency.
Care Environment Management		Identifies clinical and cost outcomes that improve safety, effectiveness, timeliness, efficiency, quality, and the degree to which they are client-centered.
		Conduct a multidisciplinary team meeting; incorporate client and/or family as part of the team meeting.

(Continued)

END-OF-PROGRAM COMPETENCIES & REQUIRED CLINICAL EXPERIENCES FOR THE CLINICAL NURSE LEADER

GRADUATE LEVEL CURRICULUM ELEMENTS	CNL ROLE FUNCTIONS	CNL ROLE EXPECTATIONS	END-OF-PROGRAM COMPETENCIES	REQUIRED CLINICAL EXPERIENCES
	Information Manager	■ Uses information systems/technologies ■ Improves health care outcomes	Uses information systems and technology at the point of care to improve health care outcomes.	Using patient information system data, design and implement a plan of care for a cohort of patients. Use aggregate data sets to prepare reports and justify needs for select care improvements. Evaluate the impact of new technologies on nursing staff, patients and families. Participate in establishing and reviewing interdisciplinary patient care plans with team.
	Systems Analyst/ Risk Anticipator	■ Participates in system reviews ■ Evaluates/anticipates client risks to improve patient safety	Participates in systems review to critically evaluate and anticipate risks to client safety to improve quality of client care delivery.	Apply evidence-based practice as basis for client care decisions. Conduct a microsystem analysis by: ■ Identifying a clinical issue with a focus on a population. ■ Conducting a trend analysis of incident reports. ■ Evaluating a sentinel event and conducting a root cause analysis (RCA). ■ Incorporating analysis of outcome data.

Clinical Outcomes Management				
				Analyzing barriers and facilitators within the organization related to the identified issue. ■ Writing an action plan related to the analysis ■ Presenting/disseminating to appropriate audience. Work with quality improvement team and engage in designing and implementing a process for improving patient safety.
Clinical Outcomes Management	Clinician	■ Designs/coordinates/evaluates care ■ Delivers care in a timely, cost effective manner ■ Emphasizes health promotion/risk reduction	Assumes accountability for health care outcomes for a specific group of clients within a unit or setting recognizing the influence of the meso- and macrosystems on the microsystem. Assimilates and applies research-based information to design, implement and evaluate client plans of care.	Plan and delegate care for clients with multiple chronic health problems, identify nursing interventions to impact outcomes of care. Using an existing database, evaluate aggregate care outcomes for a designated microsystem with focus on specific nursing interventions. Contribute to interdisciplinary plans of care based on best practice guidelines and evidence-based practice.
Clinical Outcomes Management	Outcomes Manager	■ Uses data to change practice and improve outcomes ■ Achieves optimal client outcomes	Synthesizes data, information and knowledge to evaluate and achieve optimal client and care environment outcomes.	Coordinate care for a group of patients based on desired outcomes consistent with evidence-based guidelines and quality care standards. Revise patient care based on analysis of outcomes and evidence-based knowledge. Analyze unit resources and set priorities for maximizing outcomes. Conduct a patient care team research review seminar.

(Continued)

Table AP-B.1

END-OF-PROGRAM COMPETENCIES & REQUIRED CLINICAL EXPERIENCES FOR THE CLINICAL NURSE LEADER

GRADUATE LEVEL CURRICULUM ELEMENTS	CNL ROLE FUNCTIONS	CNL ROLE EXPECTATIONS	END-OF-PROGRAM COMPETENCIES	REQUIRED CLINICAL EXPERIENCES
Clinical Outcomes Management	Educator	■ Uses teaching/ learning principles/ strategies ■ Uses current information/materials/ techniques ■ Facilitates clients learning, anticipating their health trajectory needs ■ Facilitates client care using evidence-based resources ■ Facilitates group & other health professions' learning and professional development	Uses appropriate teaching/ learning principles and strategies as well as current information, materials and technologies to facilitate the learning of clients, groups and other health care professionals.	Present a seminar or case study at a grand rounds or team meeting. Conduct health education of individual patient or cohort based on risk profile. Create or review an education module directed at patients and staff; develop a self-management guide for patients and families. Develop and implement a professional development session for other professional nursing and ancillary staff. Develop a health education plan for a unit-specific issue common to multiple clients. Implement & evaluate the health education plan, evaluating the role of the team, the teaching learning methods used, the client interactions, the expected & actual outcomes, including health status changes.

AACN CNL Implementation Task Force Members

Jolene Tornabeni, MA, RN, FACHE, FAAN *Task Force Chair*

Cynthia Flynn Capers, PhD, RN, University of Akron

Melanie Dreher, PhD, RN, FAAN, Rush University, *AACN Board liaison*

Karen Haase-Herrick, MN, RN, Northwest Organization of Nurse Executives, *AONE representative*

James Harris, DSN, RN, MBA, APRN, Chief Nursing Officer, VA Tennessee Valley Healthcare System, *VA representative*

Traci Hoiting, MS, RN, ACNP-C, Swedish Medical Center, Seattle, WA

Rose Marie Martin, BSN, RN, Arthur G. James Cancer Hospital, Columbus, OH

Judith Fitzgerald Miller, PhD, RN, FAAN, Marquette University

Charlene Connolly Quinn, PhD, RN, Department of Epidemiology and Medicine, School of Medicine University of Maryland, *Evaluation Committee Chair*

Raelene Shippee-Rice, PhD, RN, University of New Hampshire

Marcia Stanhope, DSN, RN, FAAN, University of Kentucky, *Curriculum Committee Chair*

Marge Wiggins, MBA, RN, Maine Medical Center, *Practice Model Committee Chair*

Joan Stanley, PhD, RN, CRNP, FAAN, *AACN staff liaison*

Kathy McGuinn, MSN, RN, CPHQ, *AACN staff liaison*

CNL Curriculum Committee Members

Marcia Stanhope, DSN, RN, FAAN, University of Kentucky, *Committee Chair*

Traci Hoiting, MS, RN, ACNP-C, Swedish Medical Center, Seattle, WA

Judith Fitzgerald Miller, PhD, RN, FAAN, Marquette University

Raelene Shippee-Rice, PhD, RN, University of New Hampshire

Joan Stanley, PhD, RN, CRNP, FAAN, *AACN staff liaison*

CNL Practice Model Committee Members

Marge Wiggins, MBA, RN, Maine Medical Center, *Committee Chair*

Cynthia Flynn Capers, PhD, RN, University of Akron

Melanie Dreher, PhD, RN, FAAN, Rush University

Karen Haase-Herrick, MN, RN, Northwest Organization of Nurse Executives

James Harris, DSN, RN, MBA, APRN, Chief Nursing Officer, VA Tennessee Valley Healthcare System

Rose Marie Martin, BSN, RN, Arthur G. James Cancer Hospital, Columbus, OH

Jolene Tornabeni, MA, RN, FACHE, FAAN

Kathy McGuinn, MSN, RN, CPHQ, *AACN staff liaison*

Joan Stanley, PhD, RN, CRNP, FAAN, *AACN staff liaison*

CNL Evaluation Committee Members

Charlene Connolly Quinn, PhD, RN, Department of Epidemiology and Medicine, School of Medicine University of Maryland, *Committee Chair*

Sean Clarke, PhD, RN, CRNP, CS, Center for Health Outcomes and Policy Research University of Pennsylvania, *consultant*

Sue Haddock, PhD, RN, CNAA-BC, WJB Dorn VA Hospital, *VA liaison*

Kathy Player, EdD, RN, Ken Blanchard College of Business at Grand Canyon University

Kathleen Sanford, MA, RN, DBA, FACHE, Gig Harbor Area Multicare Health System *AONE representative*

Marcia Stanhope, DSN, RN, FAAN, University of Kentucky, *Implementation TF liaison*

Jolene Tornabeni, MA, RN, FACHE, FAAN, immediate-past EVP and COO, Inova Health System, *Implementation TF liaison*

Gail Wolf, DNS, RN, UPMC Health Systems, *AONE Representative*

Joan Stanley, PhD, RN, CRNP, FAAN, *AACN staff liaison*

Kathy McGuinn, MSN, RN, CPHQ, *AACN staff liaison*

Index

AAAHC. *See* Accreditation Association for Ambulatory Health Care (AAAHC)

AACN. *See* American Association of Colleges of Nursing (AACN); American Association of Critical-Care Nurses (AACN)

AANA. *See* American Association of Nurse Anesthetists (AANA)

AANP. *See* American Academy of Nurse Practitioner (AANP)

ABNS. *See* American Board of Nursing Specialties (ABNS)

ABNSAC. *See* American Board of Nursing Specialists Accreditation Council (ABNSAC)

ABSN. *See* Accelerated Bachelor of Science in Nursing (ABSN)

Academic degrees, 1

Accelerated Bachelor of Science in Nursing (ABSN), 165

Accelerated programs, 2

Accreditation, 11, 21, 22, 33, 155

Accreditation Association for Ambulatory Health Care (AAAHC), 155

ACHNE. *See* Association of Community Health Nursing Educators (ACHNE)

ACNM. *See* American College of Nurse-Midwives (ACNM)

Acute care, 4
  CNL and, enhancement of, 67
  Doctor of Nursing programs for, 55
  hospitals, 5, 6
  institutions, 9
  nurse anesthesia programs and, 51

Advanced Clinic Access, 181

Advanced Nurse Practitioner (ANP), 18, 46, 169

Advanced Practice Nurses (APRNs), 45–47
  certification of, 4, 45, 49, 57, 81, 207
  core competencies of, 4, 207–208
  credentials of, 23–24
  doctoral degree programs for, 45–47
  educational requirements of, 4
  employment options for, 4
  interdisciplinary education of, 26
  issues related to, 9
  pharmacologic principles, understanding of, 215
  practice sites for, 4
  roles of, 195
  scope of practice of, 4, 107, 215, 263
  types of, 3–4

Advanced practice programs, 20

Advanced Practice Registered Nurses (APRNs), 142

Agency for Healthcare Research and Quality, 99

AMA. *See* American Medical Association (AMA)

American Academy of Nurse Practitioner (AANP)
  certification of, 153
  graduate programs of nursing for, 14
  history of, 20–21
  master's degree programs for, 7
  Task Force on Doctoral Preparation of Nurse Anesthetists Report, 51–52

American Association of Colleges of Nursing (AACN)
  certification by, 177
  clinical doctoral education programs for, 13
  and development of CNL, 107, 144, 175
  DNP, concerns regarding, 22